MIND
Body
MAGIC

CREATIVE ACTIVITIES
FOR ANY AUDIENCE

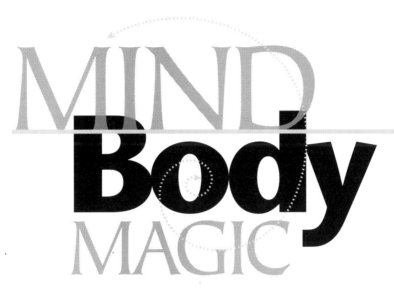

MIND Body MAGIC

CREATIVE ACTIVITIES FOR ANY AUDIENCE

MARTHA BELKNAP

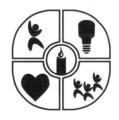

WHOLE PERSON ASSOCIATES
Duluth, Minnesota

Library of Congress Cataloging-in-Publication Data
Belknap, Martha.
    Mind-body magic / Martha Belknap.
    176 p. 23 cm.
    Includes bibliographical references.
    ISBN 1-57025-126-6 (pbk.)
    1. Exercise. 2. Mind and body. 3. Imagery (Psychology)—Therapeutic
use. 1. Title.
    RA781.B397 1997
    613.7'1—dc21   96-35696
                                                         CIP

Printed in the United States of America
10 9 8 7 6 5 4 3 2 1

WHOLE PERSON ASSOCIATES
210 W Michigan
Duluth MN 55802-1908
800-247-6789

With appreciation to

my parents, who helped me believe in myself,

my husband, who encourages my creativity,

and my students, who challenge me to expand.

Table of contents

OPENING UP OUR CREATIVITY

RELAXING INTO STILLNESS

RECOMMENDED READING

Introduction

Be who you are
Practice what you know
Teach what you learn
And continue to grow!

These words came to my mind several summers ago while I was attending a yoga and meditation retreat near Lake Tahoe. I was doing some stretches at sunrise in the woods outside my tent. Since that time, these messages have served as guidelines on many occasions, especially when I need reminders of ways to simplify my life.

My interest in teaching began in my mother's nursery school when I was four years old. My mother, Elizabeth Belknap, (who celebrated her 100th birthday this year) encouraged me to help the younger children learn skills such as tying shoelaces and zipping jackets. I was also inspired to teach by my father, Walter Belknap, whose life was dedicated to serving others. In school, I was often given opportunities to show other children what I had learned. And now, years later, I am still engaged in education, sharing with my students and friends what works in my life.

Many of the activities in this book were created in my living room while exercising, stretching, and dancing. I love discovering unusual ways to have fun while taking good care of myself. Many of the relaxation images came to me while enjoying the peace of the Colorado mountains where my husband, Bill Brennen, and I live in a home we built together. In stillness and silence my creative energies find their freedom.

I have had lots of chances to try out my ideas with the college students in my creativity classes at the University of Colorado, with parents and teachers who take my workshops, and with the participants in conference presentations. Young children, as well as the beautiful folks in my yoga classes for the elderly, have all inspired me to develop new, creative ways of moving, balancing, energizing, and relaxing.

I believe that most of us are capable of enjoying a much better quality of life than we usually experience. The following messages I keep in front of me on my desk:

Just imagine that . . .

you are smarter than you know
more courageous than you guess
stronger than you feel;
you are healthier than you are aware of
more creative than you believe
more capable than you recognize;
you are more powerful than you think
more attractive than you assume
wiser than you suppose;
you are more valuable than you have ever been told;
you are loved beyond your dreams
and you are able to make a difference
in the world that you have
not yet begun to realize.

Just imagine that!

In all my workshops and classes, I strive to create a relaxed atmosphere by emphasizing that these activities are designed to be easy, healthy, and fun! I encourage my audiences and students to open up to new experiences and allow themselves to expand in unexplored directions. I invite them to participate fully, and I also allow them to observe at times if that is their choice. I often end an activity by asking the participants to think of someone else they know who would enjoy or benefit from these experiences. I suggest that as homework, they teach the activity to their spouse, child, or friend.

I have shared variations of the activities in this book with children, teenagers, college students, parents and children together, educators, therapists, recreation directors, health professionals, couples, women's groups, the business community, and the elderly.

I encourage you as presenters, trainers, and teachers to use your creative imagination and ingenuity to adapt these activities for your own groups of various ages, walks of life, educational levels, and cultural backgrounds. As you discover effective ways to change and expand these ideas—or if you would like any guidance in that direction—I would be happy to hear from you.

Since most of these activities were originally developed for my personal enjoyment and wellness, I encourage you to experience the benefits of individual practice. Become a star without an audience, a true Mind-Body Magician!

I believe that we can inspire others most effectively by sharing our stories and by sincerely modelling in our lives what we truly believe. Above all, may you find great joy in whatever you choose to do for yourselves and for others.

Are you doing what you love?
Are you loving what you do?
Are you living who you are?
Are you loving being you?

Martha Belknap
1170 Dixon Road/Gold Hill
Boulder, CO 80302
(303) 447-9642

October 1996

STRETCHING OUR BODY/MIND

The ten activities in this section offer opportunities to experience body-mind connections from the kinesthetic perspective. Stretching is an easy, natural activity which helps us release tension from our muscles and preoccupations from our minds. The original yogis of India are believed to have developed many of their postures after observing the ways animals stretch and move. Stretching can improve circulation, strengthen breathing, relieve fatigue, reduce stiffness, release nervousness, improve flexibility, promote mental clarity, and revitalize energy.

These activities are designed to help make stretching really fun. Since many of these movements involve focusing on images of nature, they are very well suited to being enjoyed outdoors. If we pay attention to the purpose of each activity and let ourselves have a good time while we are stretching, the benefits of each movement will be greatly enhanced. Let go, laugh, allow yourself to be silly, and notice how much more relaxed and energized you feel!

River and Clouds

Balance structure with freedom
using easy t'ai chi movements.

PURPOSES
To illustrate the need for both structure and freedom.
To demonstrate the concept of physical and mental balance.
To introduce the principles of t'ai chi movement.

TIME
10–15 minutes.

MATERIALS
River and Clouds worksheet; pens or pencils.

INTRODUCTION

Westerners can learn a lot from some of the ancient traditions of the East. In Shanghai, every morning five hundred Chinese men and women, mostly elderly, practice t'ai chi in a beautiful park alongside the Whangpoo River. No one seems to be in charge but each person has a sense of when to start and what to do and how to move together perfectly!

PROCESS

Ask participants to stand up and move to the center of the room, spacing themselves an arm's length from each other. When everyone has found a relaxed position, read aloud the following script, pausing briefly after each sentence:

Imagine that you are the captain of a riverboat . . .

*Stretch your left hand out to your left side (thumb side up)
and draw it in front of your body (toward the right)
as though you were guiding a boat very carefully down a river.*

Repeat with the right hand moving from the right side to the left.

*Continue alternating hands as you affirm to yourself
that you are in charge of the direction that your boat is traveling.*

*Think about times when you need to assume responsibility
and take charge of directing your life energy . . .
(pause for 10 seconds)*

*Now stand still and imagine some white fluffy clouds in the
sky . . .*

*Reach your left hand up and across to the right
and let it drift above you (toward the left) as though a cloud
were floating by.*

Repeat with the right hand, moving from the left side to the right.

*Continue alternating hands as you remind yourself
that clouds are free to float randomly in their own directions . . .*

*Think about times when you need to release conscious control
and trust the natural flow of energy in your life . . .
(pause for 10 seconds)*

*Now coordinate these two movements together
as you imagine guiding your boat down a river
with a light cloud floating aimlessly overhead . . .*

*Moving both hands at the same time,
let one hand be the boat and one be the cloud,
switching slowly from one movement to the other . . .*

*Think about times in your life when you need to experience
both structure and freedom at the same time . . .
(pause for 10 seconds)*

Mind–Body Magic

With participants still standing, ask them to briefly share their responses to the experience by responding to the following questions:

- Were you more comfortable with one movement than the other?

- Could you stay focused on both movements simultaneously?

Ask each person to pair up with a partner to discuss the following questions. Allow 2–5 minutes for this process.

- How does this experience relate to your life?

- When would practicing this activity be helpful to you?

VARIATIONS

Distribute the **River and Clouds** worksheets. After participants have time to reflect on the applications of the metaphor in their current life, form small groups for sharing insights. Allow 5–15 minutes for participants to complete this process.

Lead the group in singing "Row, Row, Row Your Boat" and focus on the significance of each line:

Row, row, row your boat—be in control of your life
Gently down the stream—relax and go with the flow
Merrily, merrily, merrily, merrily—be joyful
Life is but a dream—let go of illusions

- Invite pairs or trios to process the messages embedded in the lyrics of this familiar song. Which theme is most important to you at this time in your life? Allow participants 3–5 minutes for discussion.

NOTES

I have found this activity of particular interest to women. They appreciate having the chance to talk about the need for balance in their lives and to share their own ways of achieving it.

When working with the elderly, I generally have my students remain seated during this activity.

©1997 Martha Belknap Whole Person Associates • 210 West Michigan • Duluth, MN 55802 • (800) 247-6789

River and Clouds

1. In what areas of your life do you need to take more control? Assume more responsibility? Actively guide your direction?

2. In what areas of your life do you need to let go and trust the flow of your natural processes?

3. In what areas of your life do you enjoy or need freedom in the context of structure?

4. In what areas of your life do you enjoy or need structure in the midst of freedom?

As Easy as ABC

Stretch your body in many different directions
using the letters of the alphabet as a guide.

PURPOSES

To release tension from the muscles.

To introduce participants to each other.

To reinforce creative movement with a memory device.

TIME

4–5 minutes.

MATERIALS

None.

PROCESS

Instruct participants to move to an open space in the room, then give the following instructions:

Stand comfortably with your arms relaxed at your sides. Check to be sure that your knees are relaxed.

We will use the letters of the alphabet to help us move in ways that are as easy as ABC. I will call out letters of the alphabet along with a movement that begins with that letter. For example, when I call out "Arching" we will link our thumbs, raise our arms overhead, and arch back. When I call out "Bending" we will reach forward toward the floor. We will continue through the alphabet, stretching with each letter.

Arching	Jumping	Swimming
Bending	Kicking	Twisting
Climbing	Leaping	Uplifting
Dancing	Moving	Vibrating
Energizing	Nodding	Walking
Flowing	Opening	eXercising
Growing	Praying	Yawning
Hugging	Quivering	Zigzagging
Ice skating	Running	

Lead participants through the exercise one more time, stretching with each letter.

After stretching through the alphabet the second time, instruct participants to pair up with a partner, preferably someone they do not know. When everyone has found a partner, give the following direction:

Spell your first name for your partner by doing a stretch that goes with each letter of your name.

VARIATIONS

Go around the group and for each successive alphabet letter, let each person in turn choose a movement that stretches a body part that begins with their letter. Other participants in the group imitate the movement. Compile a list of suggestions for each letter as you go so people have new ideas for future reference.

Choose a few letter stretches related to the group or topic and intersperse these as mnemonics to memorably demonstrate and reinforce key points during a longer workshop.

Have one person volunteer to "spell" a key word with movements for the rest of the group to guess. (e.g. words such as relax, smile, laugh, play) Or spell the name of a team, a product, or a place that is familiar to that particular group of people.

Roots and Wings

Balance different energies in your body/mind/spirit through memory, metaphor, and music.

PURPOSES
To illustrate connections between mind/body perception and energy levels.
To demonstrate the evocative nature of music.
To provide a refreshing break.

TIME
10–15 minutes.

MATERIALS
Roots and Wings worksheet; pens or pencils.

PROCESS
▨ Introduce the topic and purpose of the exercise. Give participants the following directions and then read aloud the poem, pausing after each line:

▲ Sit comfortably and close your eyes.

▲ Imagine a large tree with strong roots reaching deep down into the earth.

▲ Circling overhead, a giant bird soars on the breeze with outstretched wings.

Let your roots keep reaching downward
So your strength is ever new

Let your confidence be carried
Into everything you do

Let your wings keep reaching upward
And your spirit soar on high
Let your visions be expanded
So your dreams are free to fly!

Explain to participants that you are going to repeat the activity a second time using the same poem. Give the following instructions:

We are going to repeat the activity we just completed except this time I would like you to move to the center of the room, spacing yourself an arm's length from each other.

Take a wide stance, feet about shoulder width apart. Notice where you experience your center of gravity, and allow yourself to feel more and more grounded as that center of gravity moves lower in your body.

Ask participant to focus on their center of gravity as you read aloud the first stanza of the poem.

Let your roots keep reaching downward
So your strength is ever new
Let your confidence be carried
Into everything you do

Provide the following instructions to participants and then continue reading aloud the second stanza of the poem.

Now feel free to raise your arms and stretch on tiptoe, moving appropriately to the words of the second stanza. Be light and free as you let your center of gravity rise upward to the top of your head.

Let your wings keep reaching upward
And your spirit soar on high

Let your visions be expanded
So your dreams are free to fly!

After reading the poem a second time, distribute copies of the **Roots and Wings** worksheet to participants. Comment on how the worksheet will help them to explore the meaning of their own roots and wings. Give the following instructions:

Think about activities in your life that help you feel more grounded, centered, and in touch with your body and the earth (e.g., walking/hiking, eating cooked food such as beans and grains, gardening, working in a woodshop, dancing to drumbeats, swimming in the surf, giving or receiving a deep massage). Make a list of your activities in the column marked "Grounded" on your worksheet.

Now think about activities in your life which help you feel more uplifted, lighter, and in touch with your free spirit (e.g., sitting on a hillside at sunset, eating fruits, drinking fruit juice, practicing t'ai chi, listening to quiet music in the dark, meditating, contemplating, looking at the Milky Way). Make a list of these activities in the column marked "Uplifted" on the worksheet.

When you have finished the "Grounded" and "Uplifted" sections, complete the questions at the bottom of the worksheet.

After 8–10 minutes, divide participants into small groups and ask them to share their worksheet responses with each other.

Reconvene the entire group and conclude the session by asking participants to share any comments or insights they gained during this imagery exercise.

VARIATION

Vary this activity by playing music which is grounding and music which is uplifting, inviting participants to move to the music in two different ways. To feel grounded, I prefer music with a percussion beat and a steady rhythm. To feel uplifted, I play flute, cello, harp, and piano music with a wandering type of melody. The *adagio* movement of your favorite symphony may also be a good choice.

NOTES

Here are some suggestions for music which I enjoy moving to:

Grounding music: "Medicine Man"—Bobby McFerrin; "Prayer for the Wild Things"—Paul Winter; "Equinox"—Jean Michel Jarre; "Air on a G String"—J.S. Bach.

Uplifting music: "Inside the Great Pyramid"—Paul Horn; "Cello"—David Darling; "Peace Offering"—Alex Jones; "Gifts of the Angels"—Steven Halpern.

©1997 Martha Belknap Whole Person Associates • 210 West Michigan • Duluth, MN 55802 • (800) 247-6789

Roots and Wings

Grounded	Uplifted

1. Is there a time of day when you generally prefer grounding activities? uplifting activities?

2. How do you know when you need to be more grounded? more uplifted?

3. Do you need one type of activity more than the other? If so, why do you think this is true?

4. How do different kinds of foods affect your energy balance? Are you conscious of what you choose to eat and do to help bring your energies into balance?

Mind-Body Magic

A Trip to the Beach

*Let mental imagery
help you stretch your body.*

PURPOSES
To relax, energize, or calm a group.
To demonstrate the relaxing and energizing benefits of stretching.
To stimulate creativity.

TIME
8–10 minutes.

MATERIALS
A carpeted space in which to move and sit/lie down.

INTRODUCTION
Brain research indicates that we tend to think in images and that we respond most to perceptions that come to us through all of our senses. We also learn well through metaphors which help us make connections between one concept and another. And most of us remember better if we become actively involved in pleasurable experiences. The following activity makes use of all these principles of learning.

PROCESS
Introduce the purpose of the exercise and ask participants to move to an open space in the room an arm's length from each other. Ask them to imagine the warm sun and cool breeze on their face as they stand relaxed on a tropical beach. Lead them through the

following stretches, proceeding from one to the next, pausing briefly after each one.

Palm Tree Sway: Let your arms float overhead. Link your thumbs together and sway from side to side in the tropical breeze.

Hula Dance: Make a figure 8 movement with your hips. Let your arms move gracefully in front of you.

Coconut Roll: Let your head drop forward. Roll your head from side to side with your chin down.

Whale's Breath: Inhale deeply through your nose. Blow the air out through your mouth.

Lemonade Breath: Round your lips and make an opening in the middle. Suck air in through the hole as though you were drinking through a straw. Let the air out gently through your nose.

Turtle Stretch: Lift your shoulders up to your ears. Imagine hiding your head inside a turtle shell. Stretch your neck out slowly and look around.

Flipper Flop: Bend your elbows with your hands in front of you. Bounce your elbows against your ribs and make some dolphin sounds.

Picking Bananas: Stretch as though you were picking fruit from a tree. As you reach up with one hand, let the opposite heel lift off the ground.

Surfer's Shake: Imagine that you have just come out of the ocean. Shake the water off your hands and feet. Now dry off your back with a beach towel.

Jellyfish Float: Sit/lie down on the floor and relax completely. Take in a deep breath and let it out slowly. Feel all your tension floating away.

Gliding Gulls: Close your eyes and imagine seagulls gliding on the ocean breezes at sunset. Let your spirit be lifted up to join the flight.

Sunset Sky: Picture a glorious sunset over the ocean. Imagine seeing purple and pink, turquoise and gold in the space behind your closed eyelids. Breathe your favorite colors into your awareness.

If time allows, ask participants to share their reactions to the previous images.

VARIATIONS

You may want to do only the first nine stretches, ending with an energetic rather than a peaceful activity.

Show participants photographs of beach scenes and ask them to discuss how they feel when they are at the beach. Use the following questions to begin a discussion:

What kind of beach do you enjoy the most?

Do you feel a different kind of energy near the ocean? near a lake? along a river? near a waterfall?

How does the presence of moving water affect you?

Stretch to Infinity

*Stretch your body in a variety of directions
using the infinity symbol as a pattern for movement.*

PURPOSES
To expand consciousness of inner self and outer potential.
To build camaraderie in small groups.
To foster a sense of connectedness with the universe and the infinite.

TIME
3–5 minutes.

MATERIALS
None.

INTRODUCTION
  The infinity symbol is one which most of us enjoyed learning
to draw when we were children. That same pattern is used in many
activities such as auto racing, horsemanship, and figure skating.
Think about how our ability to learn and our capacity to develop
are essentially unlimited and boundless. As human beings we have
infinite potential for growth and change!

PROCESS
  Introduce the exercise and ask participants to stand up, allowing themselves plenty of room for them to move freely. Read aloud
the following script, pausing briefly after each line:

> *Stand comfortably with your arms relaxed at your sides
> and your knees unlocked.*

Close your eyes.

Imagine the infinity symbol . . . or a figure 8 . . . lying on its side.
Imagine that symbol curving around your feet.

Open your eyes and begin to move
so your knees trace that figure 8 pattern.
Now let your hips begin to move in the same direction.
Trace a figure 8 in the air behind you with your tailbone.
And now in front of you with your belly button.

Focus your attention into your right thumb
and begin to trace a figure 8 in the air next to your upper leg.
Now move your wrist . . . and your elbow . . .
and your shoulder in the same pattern.
Let your whole arm move in a swooping motion
in front of your body and then behind you.

Continue to see the shape of the infinity symbol in your
imagination.
Now let your right arm relax at your side.

Focus your attention into your left thumb
and begin to move it in a figure 8 pattern.
Include your wrist . . . your elbow . . .
your shoulder . . . and your whole arm.
Now link your two thumbs together and move both arms
at once.
With your eyes open and your head still,
follow the pattern of your arms with your eyes.
Then let your arms relax at your sides.

Close your eyes and imagine an infinity symbol in front of
your face.
Trace it with the tip of your nose.
Let the pattern get larger and larger.

Now imagine a ray of light coming out the top of your head

and trace a figure 8 on the ceiling above you.
Bring your head to rest.
With your eyes still closed, trace the same figure with your eyes.
And now do it with the bottom of your chin.
Keep your head still and repeat the movement with your chin and jaw.
Can you do it with your tongue?

Open your eyes and begin to move your entire body in a figure 8 pattern.
Go horizontally for awhile and then vertically.
Feel yourself reaching out to infinity.
Face another person
and let your swirling arms send energy all around your partner . . . up and down . . . around the waist . . . around the knees . . . over the head.
Join another group of two and continue this movement with four people in a circle . . .
and then with eight.
Keep eye contact with the people to whom you are sending energy.
Notice the energy that you are receiving.

Conclude the exercise by reading the following poem. Encourage participants to reflect on the infinite potential each of us has.

I move from this moment, this time, and this place,
And reach from this room into infinite space
I feel the vibrations from Venus and Mars,
And send out my light to the infinite stars.

VARIATION

Ask participants to discuss how they feel about the concept of infinite potential.

I Bow to the Earth

Stretch your body with simple yoga
movements using familiar images of nature.

PURPOSES
To teach basic yoga techniques.
To introduce an easy daily self-care ritual.
To get acquainted nonverbally with other participants.

TIME
3–5 minutes.

MATERIALS
Poster of images and corresponding movements for display and easy reference during the stretch.

INTRODUCTION
Yoga is a Sanskrit work meaning union. From the same root comes the English word yoke as in a yoke of oxen. I see the practice of yoga as a way of promoting a union between the conscious mind and the physical body, between the individual soul and the universal spirit. Hatha Yoga involves stretching and balancing postures, deep breathing, and quiet relaxation. My favorite saying about yoga is that it is designed to "make our bodies sing but not scream." Yoga can also be seen as a key to unlocking the treasure chest within ourselves. It can be a way of bringing ourselves into a state of better balance and flexibility, of greater vitality and inner peace.

PROCESS

▦ Introduce the purpose of the exercise and explain that we will be repeating the same images of nature and movements four different times, each time in a slightly different way.

▦ Give participants the following instruction before you read the list of images and movements aloud the first time:

▲ Stand in a comfortable relaxed position with your arms at your sides and your knees slightly bent. Follow me as I suggest some images of nature to which we can move:

Images	Movements
I bow to the earth	bend forward from the waist reaching your hands toward the earth
I lift to the sky	reach up with both arms stretched over head
I reach for the sun	open your arms to the side as though you were embracing the sun
And the clouds on high	let your hands float from side to side overhead
I welcome the rain	lower your arms to the side to waist level as you move your fingers like falling rain
That flows to the sea	reach your arms out to the sides as you swing around, imitating ocean waves
I honor the spirit	bring palms together in front of your chest
In you and in me	extend your arms outward with palms up and then cross hands with palms touching chest

Mind–Body Magic

After completing the list, repeat the sequence a second time. Ask participants to say the verse with you as you all move together.

With each image, prompt with key words of the corresponding movement.

To complete the sequence the third time, ask participants to turn, face someone near them, and make eye contact. Request that participants do this stretch together with their partner. Encourage participants to look directly at each other, especially on the last two lines.

For the fourth and final time, ask participants to turn around and become partners with someone else.

Ask participants to sit down and conclude the session by asking for their feedback and reactions.

NOTES

I especially like to do this activity with young children and their parents. Also this is one of the favorite activities in my yoga classes for the elderly.

Where in the World?

*Gently stretch your body/mind
using seven images from nature.*

PURPOSES
To provide focus at the beginning of a session.
To provide closure at the end of a session.
To introduce the power of imagery.

TIME
4–5 minutes.

MATERIALS
None.

PROCESS

▨ Ask group members to move to the center of the room an arm's length from each other. Encourage them to find a relaxed standing position and lead them through the following guided imagery:

Desert at Dawn: With your arms relaxed at your sides, move your hands as though you were smoothing the warm sand on the desert. Sway gently from side to side as your hands move around your body.

A Roaring River: Lift your arms to the side at waist level and imagine a river flowing around you as your hands become the rapids in the swift current.

The Surf is Up!: Lift your arms to the side at shoulder level and imagine the ocean waves rolling into shore as your hands become the breakers crashing on the beach around you.

Mountains at Mid-day: Lift your arms overhead and trace the outline of your favorite mountain range covered with huge drifts of fresh snow.

Foothills and Valleys: Lower your arms to shoulder level as you let your hands find their way through the forests in the foothills and into the valleys below.

Wind in the Wheat Fields: Lower your arms to waist level as you let your hands move like the wind through the wheat fields and over the rolling farmlands.

A Lake in the Moonlight: With your arms relaxed at your sides, move your hands as though they were gliding over the surface of a quiet lake. Close your eyes and sway very slowly, breathing in the silence and the stillness of the moonlight.

If time allows, encourage participants to reflect on the images from nature. Lead a closing discussion using the following question:

Which image was the most tranquil to you? Why?

VARIATION

Show photographs of a desert, river, ocean, mountain, etc. Ask participants to share which geographical area is most familiar and comfortable to them.

What elements of the scene help you feel at ease there?

Do you feel a different energy at different elevations?

What area would you like to visit more often?

L–O–V–E Stretch

*Recharge your body/mind/spirit as
you stretch and relax to an affirming acronym.*

PURPOSES
To help people open up.
To promote self-esteem.
To build group spirit.

TIME
3–5 minutes.

MATERIALS
L–O–V–E Stretch worksheets; pens or pencils.

PROCESS
▪ Introduce the topic and ask participants to move to an open space in the room where they can move freely. Read aloud the following script:

Stand in a comfortable position with your arms at your sides and your knees relaxed.

Think of the four letters in the word LOVE as we do this stretch together.

First letter—L —Let in the Light

Lift your arms to the sides with palms upturned.

Reach your arms upward as you invite the light of the sun to come into your being.

Look upward toward the sky.

Mind–Body Magic

Lower your hands in front of your face
as though you were bathing your face with sunshine.

Let in the light.

Second letter—O—be Open to Opportunities

Reach your arms out in front of your body with palms up.
Open your arms to the sides at waist level.
Rotate from side to side reaching out for all the opportunities that
are around you
Opportunities for friendship, beauty, joy, health, peace.
What other opportunities are there for you?
Be open to opportunities.

Next letter—V—Vibrate with Vitality

With your arms at your sides,
begin to shake your body in whatever way feels good to you.
Feel vibrations of energy moving through your whole body.
Move your seat, your hips, your knees.
Imagine a current energizing your whole being with vitality.
Feel the vibrations moving from head to toe.
Let yourself come alive!
Vibrate with vitality.

Last letter—E—Experience Ease

As you close your eyes and breathe in,
lift your arms, palms down, up to waist level.
As you breathe out, lower your arms
and let yourself experience ease.
Inhale and lift . . . exhale and release.
Inhale and lift . . . exhale and release.
Experience ease.

Repeat the actions from the beginning, asking participants to say the following words along with you:

L—I let in the light
O—I am open to opportunities
V—I vibrate with vitality
E—I experience ease.

Ask participants to return to their seats and lead a closing discussion on the importance of recharging your body/mind/spirit.

VARIATION

After reading aloud the guided imagery script, distribute a copy of the **L–O–V–E Stretch** worksheets to each participant. Form small groups of 4–6 participants and encourage them to share their responses with each other.

NOTES

I particularly like to do this activity with the elderly, with couples, and with groups which meet around Valentine's Day.

©1997 Martha Belknap • Whole Person Associates • 210 West Michigan • Duluth, MN 55802 • (800) 247-6789

L–O–V–E *Stretch*

L—Let in the light

My typical sources of light, inspiration, or truth are:

_____

_____

_____

One new light or energy source I would like to let in is:

_____

_____

_____

O—Open to opportunities

The most intriguing opportunities I can see in my life right now are: _____

_____

_____

One new opportunity I am ready to pursue is: _____

_____

_____

_____

©1997 Martha Belknap Whole Person Associates • 210 West Michigan • Duluth, MN 55802 • (800) 247-6789

L–O–V–E Stretch (continued)

V—Vibrate with vitality

My usual sources of energy and vitality are:

One part of my life which needs a vitality boost these days is:

E—Experience ease

The most peaceful place in my life is:

I feel most at ease when:

One way I need to find more peace or be more at ease is:

Glad to Be Me

Celebrate the body/mind/spirit
with a verse and visualization.

PURPOSES
To provide an experience of self-affirmation.
To promote trust and self-respect.

TIME
4–5 minutes.

MATERIALS
None.

PROCESS
░ Introduce the topic and purpose of the exercise. Give participants the following directions, then read the script slowly, pausing briefly after each line:

⊿ Stand comfortably with your knees slightly bent and your arms relaxed at your sides.

⊿ Close your eyes and listen to the following verse as you visualize these images of nature:

I'm a plant that is growing
I'm a stream that is flowing
I'm an eagle on high
Lifting up to the sky
I'm the breeze that is blowing
I'm the sun that is glowing

I'm the waves of the sea
I am glad to be me!

Now ask participants to put the following creative movements to each of the images as you read the verse aloud again:

plant:	place palms together in front of the chest and reach up and out to the sides like branches
stream:	extend the arms outward at waist level and rotate the body from side to side moving the arms like a flowing current
eagle:	extend the arms upward and lift them overhead moving the arms like wings
breeze:	move the arms back and forth in a wavelike motion in front of the body
sun:	extend the arms overhead and reach out to the sides like rays of light
waves:	rotate one hand around the other in front of the body like rolling surf
me:	reach overhead and draw the hands down in front of the body and then point the hands toward the feet

Ask participants to select a partner. Instruct them to repeat the stretch facing each other as you say the verse out loud a third time.

Ask participants to turn around and repeat the stretch with a new partner as you read the verse aloud one final time.

VARIATION

When I do this activity with children I add the following two lines to the verse:

I'm a song without end
I am glad you're my friend

I encourage the children to create the movements that are appropriate to go with these words or you can teach them the following movements to the verse using American Sign Language:

song: extend the left hand and point the fingertips of the right hand toward the left palm as you wave the right arm back and forth (like conducting music)

without end: Combine the signs for always and still (see below)

always: make a clockwise circle in front of you with the index finger

still: make the letter Y with the thumb and little finger extended and move the hand forward with the palm facing down

glad: pat both hands on the chest a few times with an upward motion (like lifting your heart)

friend: hook the two index fingers together, right over left, then left over right (like a close link)

NOTES

Recently when I was teaching this activity in my yoga class for the elderly, one of my students who is 96 years old—a former school teacher—pointed out that grammatically speaking, the last line should be "I'm glad to be I." Then she was quick to add that poetically speaking, "I'm glad to be me" fits the rhyme scheme better.

Good Morning Sun, Good Evening Moon

Stretch, breathe, and relax
to the comforting image of daily cycles.

PURPOSES
To help people draw energy inward for focusing and centering.
To provide an experience of connecting creativity with images and needs.
To quiet down after conflict or emotional moments.

TIME
4–5 minutes.

MATERIALS
None.

PROCESS
▨ Introduce the topic and purposes of the exercise to participants. Give them the following instructions, then read the poem slowly, pausing briefly after each line:

  ▴ Stand with your arms relaxing comfortably at your sides and your knees slightly bent.

  ▴ As you listen to the following verse, picture the sun and the moon sending light and energy down to the earth:

  Welcome the sun shining bright
  Filling us with healing light

Welcome the moon high above
Filling us with healing love.

Ask participants to begin to move their arms and breathe in time with each line as you read it aloud again. Give them the following instructions:

- First line: Inhale and lift your outstretched arms up the sides of your body until they are reaching overhead with palms facing each other.

- Second line: Exhale and lower your hands down the front of your body with palms facing you.

- Third line: Inhale and lift your hands up the front of your body until they are reaching overhead.

- Fourth line: Open your arms and lower them down the sides of your body until they are hanging loosely at rest.

Encourage participants to repeat these movements as you say the verse out loud again. Make the following comments:

- As you listen to the first two lines, imagine drawing in the warmth and glow of the sunlight.

- As you listen to the last two lines, imagine drawing in the coolness and clarity of the moonlight.

Conclude the exercise by asking participants to share any additional comments or insights they learned from this activity.

VARIATION

These verses can also be sung to the tune of:

"We are the flow, we are the ebb,
We are the weavers, we are the web"

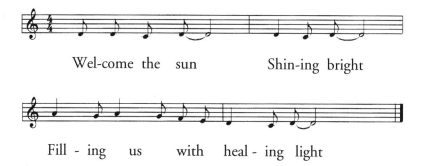

Wel-come the sun   Shin-ing bright

Fill - ing   us   with   heal - ing light

NOTES

I especially like to do these stretches in a quiet place outdoors at dawn and dusk.

Some other affirmations regarding the sun and the moon include:

I invite the *light* of the sun to awaken my *mind*.

I breathe in the *energy* of the sun to enliven my *body*.

I allow the *warmth* of the sun to open my *heart*.

I draw in the *radiance* of the sun to uplift my *soul*.

I invite the *light* of the moon to quiet my *mind*.

I breathe in the *energy* of the moon to relax my *body*.

I allow the *magic* of the moon to still my *heart*.

I let the *silence* of the moon bring peace to my *soul*.

Mind–Body Magic

ACTIVATING OUR ENERGY

The ten activities in this section offer opportunities to experience body-mind connections from the energy perspective. Energy is known by different terms in various systems and cultures. In the Indian tradition of yoga, which is about 5,000 years old, the vital life force is called *prana*. Acupuncture and acupressure refer to the Chinese word *chi* as in t'ai chi. The Japanese healing arts and martial arts use the term *ki* as found in aikido.

This vital energy is found in the air we breathe, the food we eat, the water we drink, the thoughts we think. When tensions and toxins accumulate in our systems, they block the natural flow of healthy energy which circulates through the meridians of our bodies. For many people, healing is the process of releasing those blocks and providing clear channels so the life force can move more freely. The following activities are designed to help bring movement and massage into our experience, thus activating our energy and helping to promote more balance, vitality, and freedom in our lives.

Pledge of Allegiance to Fun

*Promote laughter and set the stage for
having fun together as you playfully make the pledge.*

PURPOSES

To start a workshop or presentation on a lively note.
To enliven the group when energy is starting to wane.
To close a session on humor as a stress management skill.

TIME

1–2 minutes.

MATERIALS

Duplicated copies of the Pledge to distribute later (optional).

INTRODUCTION

Medical research indicates that laughter really is good medicine. People with a good sense of humor tend to live longer, healthier lives. Many people find that a hearty laugh acts as a natural painkiller. Laughter involves the energetic movement of the lungs, heart, belly, and other organs, which thus receive a beneficial internal massage. Happy facial expressions can increase the blood flow to the brain, which then releases chemicals affecting the immune system in a positive way. I love the reminder that we need a good laugh-ative every day in order to promote reg-hilarity!

PROCESS

Ask participants to stand in a relaxed position and give them the following directions:

- Place your right hand over your heart.

- Place your left index finger on someone else's nose.

Make sure fingers and noses are in place. Read the Pledge aloud and instruct participants to repeat each line after you.

I pledge allegiance to the fun
of the Uplifting States of Amusement
and to the playfulness for which it stands,
celebration, filled with joy irrepressible
with liberty and laughter for all!

- Change partners and repeat the activity.

- Change partners once more and repeat the Pledge using a funny voice or a silly face.

VARIATION

Ask the group to share ways they play and enjoy humor. Generate a long list. Then solicit reasons why people don't play as much as they would like to. Make a list of these obstacles to play. Divide into teams and create additional pledges to playfulness that fit the audience and setting.

NOTES

Formal groups might require extra warm-up time and perhaps some coaxing to get involved. If there is a "boss" in the group, use that person to demonstrate the proper technique of finger-to-nose. When the boss is willing to be silly, others are more likely to go along.

O Great Spirit

*Balance and energize your body
using images from Native American culture.*

PURPOSES
To identify areas for personal exploration and growth.
To illustrate insights available from other cultures.
To explore spirituality as a wellness component.

TIME
4–5 minutes.

MATERIALS
O Great Spirit worksheet; pens or pencils.

INTRODUCTION
░ In many native traditions, Spirit is seen as a balance between father and mother energies, male and female qualities, god and goddess figures. Unfortunately in many other traditions the feminine has been lost, disregarded, or assigned a lesser importance. This activity helps us to bring both the male and female concepts of Spirit back into balance.

PROCESS
░ Introduce the activity and ask participants to move to an open space in the room where they can move freely. Give the following instructions:

░ Stand comfortably with your arms relaxed at your sides and your knees slightly bent.

Close your eyes and listen as I slowly read the following verse:

O Great Spirit, Father of the Sky,
Lift up our wings and teach us how to fly
O Great Spirit, Mother of our Birth,
Teach us to walk more gently on the earth
O Great Spirit, Brother of the Air,
Teach us to feel thy presence everywhere
O Great Spirit, Sister of the Sea,
Teach us to live in peace and harmony

Explain to participants that you will read the verses again and that this time, as they listen to the lines, they should move slowly to each of these images, using the movements you demonstrate:

Words	Movements
O Great Spirit	palms together in front of chest
Father of the Sky	open arms overhead
Lift up our wings	move arms up and down
and teach us how to fly	like wings of a bird
O Great Spirit	palms together in front of chest
Mother of our Birth	extend arms down toward the earth
Teach us to walk	walk in small circle clockwise
more gently on the earth	with arms extended to the side
O Great Spirit	palms together in front of chest
Brother of the Air	lift arms up to the side
Teach us to feel	move outstretched arms overhead
thy presence everywhere	from side to side
O Great Spirit	palms together in front of chest
Sister of the Sea	extend arms forward, palms up
Teach us to live	walk in a small circle
In peace and harmony	counterclockwise with arms extended

Repeat this activity several times saying the words out loud as you lead participants through the motions.

VARIATIONS

These words may also be sung to the tune of the Native American chant:

O Great Spirit
Earth, Sun, Sky and Sea
You are within
And all around me

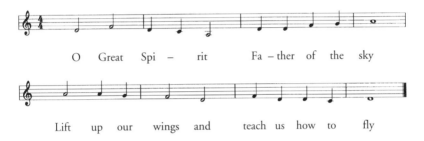

Distribute the **O Great Spirit** worksheet to participants to help them explore personal applications of the verse. When the worksheet is completed, ask participants to form small groups to share their insights and resolutions.

Ask participants to divide into pairs or trios to create chants or songs that affirm spiritual truths, wishes for well-being, expressions of hope or need. Encourage them to devise appropriate movements to accompany the message.

©1997 Martha Belknap   Whole Person Associates   •   210 West Michigan   •   Duluth, MN 55802   •   (800) 247-6789

O Great Spirit

Father
What helps you feel uplifted?
In what ways are you unable to soar?

Brother
What helps you feel the
presence of spirit?
In what ways are you out of
touch with spirit?

Sister
What helps you live in peace?
In what ways are you out
of harmony?

Mother
What helps you feel connected to the earth?
In what ways could you walk more gently?

Chakra Massage

Stimulate the seven energy centers of the body.

PURPOSES

To introduce alternative concepts of mind/body.

To provide an energizing transition in the middle of a long session.

To teach mind/body self-care skills.

TIME

3–5 minutes.

MATERIALS

None.

INTRODUCTION

In the study of yoga there are numerous energy pathways in the human body which intersect at seven major energy centers called *chakras*, a Sanskrit word meaning *wheel*. These seven centers extend from the base of the spine to the top of the head. They have been associated with the seven colors of the spectrum and with the seven tones of the musical scale. Each chakra is related to the functioning of specific glands and organs of the body. They are also thought to relate to basic human needs such as security, intimacy, power, love, creativity, awareness, and communion.

PROCESS

Introduce the topic and ask participants to move to an open space in the room where they can move freely. Slowly read the following script aloud:

Stand in a comfortable position with your arms at your sides and your knees relaxed.

The first chakra is at the base of the spine.
Make fists with both hands and gently rap on the area around your tailbone.
Move your fists up and down the lower part of the spine.
Give yourself a loving massage all around your seat.

The second chakra is in the abdomen.
Using both fists gently rap on your belly in a circular motion going up on the left side and down on the right.
You are following the direction in which food is digested.
Feel yourself energizing this lower part of your body.

The third chakra is at the solar plexus.
With bent elbows begin to flap your arms against the sides of your ribcage to energize the central part of your body.
Now shift your weight from one foot to the other and make some noise.
Move around the room and let yourself be silly.
Be sure to laugh at yourself and at others!

The fourth chakra is at the heart.
Using both fists gently pound on your chest.
Stimulate the area around your heart and lungs.
Move up to the top of your chest on either side.
Now make some Tarzan sounds to go along with this activity!

The fifth chakra is at the throat.
With one hand gently massage the front of your neck near the base of the throat.
You may find it more comfortable to use two hands around the back of the neck,
reaching your fingers along the cervical vertebrae and up toward the base of the brain.

The sixth chakra is between the eyebrows.
Lean forward slightly
and place your two thumbs between your eyebrows
with your open palms facing up
and your fingers resting on your head.
Use your thumbs to massage that area
and bring extra energy there.
Imagine that you can iron out the frown lines
that may be present from time to time.

The seventh chakra is at the crown of the head.
Use your fingertips
and gently tap the top of your head like raindrops.
Move around in all directions.
Now do the same thing with gentle fists.
Give yourself a shampoo using your fingertips to scrub
your scalp.
Also rub your ears vigorously with the palms of your hands.
This helps to stimulate pressure points
related to many different nerves in the body.
Feel yourself being energized and rejuvenated.

Now reverse the process
starting with the massage of the head and proceeding down
to the eyebrows . . .
the throat . . .
the heart . . .
the solar plexus . . .
the abdomen . . .
the base of the spine.

Now shake your arms and legs
and let yourself feel energy moving freely to all parts of
your body.

Lift your arms in the air,
dance around the room
and share this joyful energy with others.

Ask participants to take their seats, and conclude the exercise by encouraging them to briefly share their experiences with others in the group.

VARIATION

Form groups of 2–3 participants and ask them to reflect on what they experienced. Reconvene the entire group and lead a discussion by using the following questions:

Which chakra felt most in need of stimulation?

What feelings do you associate with the different chakra areas?

Where do you typically experience energy flow and blockage in your body?

Auto/Body Check-Up

*Use the care of your car as a metaphor
for the care of your body/mind.*

PURPOSES
To expand awareness of personal self-care.
To make specific plans for changes in lifestyle.
To share personal suggestions with others.

TIME
15–20 minutes.

MATERIALS
Auto/Body Check-Up worksheets; pens or pencils.

INTRODUCTION
We know that both our cars and our bodies perform better when we practice regular preventive maintenance. We would be in deep trouble (and debt!) if we raced our cars too hard, neglected regular care and tune-ups, and then had to have our cars towed into the repair shop. Are there times when we treat our personal vehicles, our bodies, in a similar way?

PROCESS
Introduce the subject matter and ask participants to pair up with a partner. One at a time, read aloud the following questions, asking participants to share their answers with their partner.

If you were a automobile, what kind would you be?

- What would you look like?

- How fast would you go?

- What condition would you be in?

- Is there a relationship between the car you currently drive and the kind of person you are?

- In what ways are the energies similar?

Distribute the **Auto/Body Check-Up** worksheets to participants. As they complete it, ask them to pay particular attention to their attitudes toward caring for their car and toward caring for their body.

After everyone has finished with the worksheet, form groups of 3–4 participants. Ask them to discuss the following questions:

- What did you observe about yourself?

- Did you notice anything surprising?

Reconvene the entire group and ask participants to share any additional comments or insights they gained during this activity.

NOTES

When I use this activity with teenagers, I begin by having them close their eyes and picture their dream car—the make and model, the year, the color, the accessories, the interior, and who is sitting next to them in the passenger's seat!

Auto/Body Check-Up

Fuel

The fuel I need for my car is:

❏ regular   ❏ lead-free   ❏ supreme   ❏ diesel

The fuels I need more of for my body are:

❏ fresh vegetables   ❏ other foods such as
❏ meat/fish/poultry/eggs
❏ fresh fruits/juices
❏ beans/nuts/seeds
❏ whole grains/cereals
❏ dairy products

Fluids

I use _____ oil in my car and need to keep it clean with regular oil changes.

I need to keep my blood clean by checking my intake of:

❏ sugar   ❏ salt   ❏ fats   ❏ caffeine   ❏ alcohol   ❏ drugs

Air

I need to put about _____ pounds of air pressure in my tires.

I need to regulate the air in my lungs by checking my intake of:

❏ nicotine   ❏ smoke   ❏ smog   ❏ fumes   ❏ dust   ❏ pollen

Body Work

To improve its appearance, my car needs:

❏ washing   ❏ waxing   ❏ vacuuming   ❏ body repairs

To improve my appearance and hygiene, I need to check my:

❏ skin   ❏ hair   ❏ nails   ❏ teeth
❏ posture   ❏ breath   ❏ body odor ❏ weight

©1997 Martha Belknap Whole Person Associates • 210 West Michigan • Duluth, MN 55802 • (800) 247-6789

Auto/Body Check-Up *(continued)*

Maintenance

My engine needs a regular tune-up to check the:

❏ points   ❏ filter   ❏ timing   ❏ brakes

❏ battery   ❏ alignment   ❏ plugs/condenser

My body/mind needs a balance of rest and activity which I can achieve by providing more:

❏ sleep/relaxation   ❏ massage/physical contact

❏ exercise/stretching   ❏ mental stimulation

❏ deep breathing   ❏ creative self-expression

❏ laughter/fun/play   ❏ companionship/love

❏ solitude/silence   ❏ affection/sex

❏ time alone with nature ❏ meditation/prayer

Observations

1. In looking over the maintenance requirements for my car and observing how carefully I attend to them, I would say that my style of caring for my car is:

2. In looking over the maintenance requirements for my body and observing how carefully I attend to them, I would say that my style of caring for my body/mind is:

3. I am ready to begin taking better care of myself by making the following change:

Mind-Body Magic

Weather Report

Release tension in the neck, shoulders, and
upper back by using familiar images of weather.

PURPOSES
To teach simple massage skills.
To enhance a presentation on workplace self-care skills.
To provide a relaxation break.

TIME
10–12 minutes.

MATERIALS
None.

INTRODUCTION
Massage is an ancient healing art as well as a special form of communication between people. Appropriate human touch based on trust and caring can promote the flow of healing energy, enhance relaxation, and bring relief from muscular tension and pain. There are many ways that we can help each other come into balance mentally and physically through the use of simple massage techniques. The following activity is designed to be done in a classroom setting, at the workplace, at home, or anywhere that feels appropriate to you.

PROCESS
Introduce the topic and purpose of the exercise and give participants the following instructions:

▲ Pair up with a partner and find a spot in the room where you have space to move.

▲ One partner should sit cross-legged on the floor. The other person will kneel down and place their hands comfortably on their partner's shoulders from behind.

▲ As I read aloud the following weather report, I will lead you through a tension-relieving massage. During the Weather Report, check to be sure that your partner is comfortable and enjoying the activity. Adjust the amount of pressure you are applying, if necessary. Let's get started:

Begin by tapping your fingers lightly along the top of your partner's shoulders.

*Extend these gently falling **snowflakes** up the back of the neck to the top of the head.*

*Change the snowflakes into **raindrops**, tapping a little harder on the head, neck, and shoulders.*

*Let the raindrops become **hailstones**, flicking your wrists as you let your fingertips bounce a little harder. Check with your partner to find out what amount of pressure feels OK.*

*Now create some **thunder**. Cup your hands and clap them across the shoulders and down along the top of the arms.*

*Next comes the **lightning**. Use the sides of your hands with a chopping motion against the shoulders and upper back.*

*Use your thumbs like the eye of a **tornado**. Press into the muscles with small deep circles. Find out where your partner would like the tornado to land.*

*Now for the **meteor shower**. Make fists and pound up and down the back on either side of the spinal column.*

*We are about to have a **blizzard**. Move your fingertips vigorously around the upper back and shoulders. Imagine snow and wind being blown together up and down the mountainside.*

*Prepare for the **earthquake**. Hold onto your partner's upper arms and gently shake the whole upper body.*

*Get ready for the **tidal wave**. Place your palms on the upper back and move them vigorously from the shoulders down to the waist. Imagine waves sloshing up and down the coast.*

Now the storm is over. Feel the calm as you place your hands gently on the shoulders and rest. Send warmth into the muscles as you imagine soothing energy flowing out of your hands into your partner's body.

*Visualize a beautiful **rainbow** spanning the sky. Feel the peace and serenity of this quiet scene. Very gradually, lift your hands several inches above your partner's shoulders. Hold them there for a few seconds. Then lower your hands to your sides and shake them gently.*

After the massage is finished, instruct participants to change places with their partner and repeat the activity.

Lead a closing discussion using the following questions:

What was the most soothing part of the massage?

Which area of your body seemed to hold the most tension?

How can you relax that part of your body?

VARIATIONS

In small groups brainstorm your typical tension spots and create metaphors for a relaxing massage of those areas.

You may want to present the Weather Report like an ongoing travelog and introduce the weather conditions which are specific to various parts of the country. For example, a snowstorm in Colorado, a thunderstorm in Minnesota, a tornado in Kansas, an earthquake in California, a tidal wave in Hawaii.

NOTES

When working with active children we need to make sure that they are being considerate of one another. I often suggest that they are giving a gift to their partners. In a while the gift will be returned to them. Ask them how they can offer the gift in such a way that it will be enjoyed, appreciated, and then returned to them as they would like. I also suggest that they go home and offer to become "weathermen" for their parents and grandparents.

In one of my classes in a summer enrichment program for gifted children, I was teaching simple shoulder and back massage techniques to a group of twelve- to fifteen-year-old boys and girls. At first I was a little uneasy about how these adolescents would handle a potentially embarrassing situation. I started by presenting the information in a very straightforward manner with clear basic instructions. The children were mature enough to respond very appropriately. When I asked them to change places with their partners for the second round, I added, "You handled that so well I would like to enhance the mood a little. We'll turn the lights down and play some quiet music." One of the boys who had received a massage in the first group said, "Is that fair? They are going to get the gourmet treatment, and we only received the generic variety!"

Mind-Body Magic

Give Your Face a Lift

Stimulate and relax the
muscles of the face and head.

PURPOSES

To demonstrate the need to release accumulated tension.

To teach self-care techniques.

To provide a short relaxation break.

TIME

5–10 minutes.

MATERIALS

None.

INTRODUCTION

Acupressure is a form of massage in which specific points on the body are stimulated to increase the flow of blood and open up the channels of energy. Shiatsu, a Japanese form of acupressure, comes from the word *shi* meaning fingers and *atsu* meaning pressure. One advantage of this technique is that it can easily be done on your own face.

PROCESS

Introduce the exercise and ask participants to think about suggestions for handling difficult situations in life. Give the group these examples:

Keep a stiff upper lip.

Keep your nose to the grindstone.

Keep your eyes peeled.
Keep your chin up.
Grit your teeth.
Grin and bear it.
Bite the bullet.
Prick up your ears.

░ Solicit other examples of kinesthetic expressions from the group. No wonder many of us carry signs of stress around our faces!

░ Explain to participants that we are going to do an exercise that will stimulate and relax the muscles of the face and head. Make sure each person is sitting down. Read the following script aloud, pausing after each line:

Let's practice some ways to let go of that tension.
Sit in a comfortable position with your spine straight.
After each one of these stretches,
rest a moment and take a deep breath.
Let the air out slowly
as you feel energy flowing into your face.
Imagine that you can breathe out through your closed eyelids,
your cheeks, and your chin.

Tilt your head back slowly,
stretch your chin up,
and press your lower lip toward your nose.

Open your mouth slightly
and slide your jaw and lower lip from side to side.

Open your mouth wide
and say the vowels of the alphabet A-E-I-O-U out loud
as you exaggerate the stretch with each letter.
Repeat several times.

Close your lips and blow up your cheeks with air.

Push the air back and forth from one side to the other
as though you were using mouthwash.

Imagine that your face is like a wrinkled prune.
Squeeze your eyes together, purse your lips,
and pull all the muscles of your face toward the end of your nose.

Tilt your head back slightly,
open your eyes wide, and stick out your tongue.
Reach your tongue toward your chin and then toward your nose.

Imagine that a fly has landed on the end of your nose.
Try to get it off without using your hands.
Wiggle your nose in all directions.
Pretend the fly is on your forehead . . . on your cheek . . .
the other cheek . . . and on your chin.
Now the fly has flown away, and you can relax your face.

Imagine that you have a big wad of chewing gum in your mouth.
Chew it on one side . . . and then on the other.
Chomp down very hard as you chew.

Imagine that your face is made of rubber.
Use your hands to press your cheeks up toward your eyes.
Push your face muscles around in all directions
and make yourself look like an ugly monster.

Pinch the bridge of your nose
and massage the area between your eyebrows.

Rub your palms together and create some warmth in your hands.
Place your palms gently over your closed eyelids.
Feel yourself sending relaxing energy into your eyelids
and into the muscles around your eyes.
Notice what colors are visible to you.
Imagine that you can see into the darkness behind your
closed eyes.

With your eyes still closed,
use your fingers to massage the rest of your face:
Use your middle fingers to press on the outside of your nostrils
as you make small circles.
Pinch your eyebrows with your thumbs and index fingers
moving from the bridge of your nose to your temples several times.
Use your index and middle fingers to make small circles at
your temples.
Reverse the direction of the circles.

Squeeze the tops of your ears and pull up.
Pinch your earlobes but do not pull down
as that tends to deplete your energy.
Slide your middle fingers up and down in front of your ears
while you move your index fingers up and down behind your ears.
Apply as much pressure as is comfortable.
Use the palms of your hands and rub your ears very briskly.

Reach around to the back of your head
and massage the area at the top of your neck
near the base of your brain.

Hold onto the tops of your shoulders near your neck
and give yourself a firm massage.
Squeeze your shoulder muscles together while you are
doing this.

Now relax your hands in your lap
and feel the energy in your head, neck, and shoulders.
Is there any place that needs a little more attention?
With your eyes closed,
let your eyes roll up toward the top of your head like marbles.
Relax your jaw and let your cheeks be loose.
Let the tip of your tongue rest against the top of your mouth.
Listen to your quiet breathing . . .
in and out through your nose.

You may want to add a quiet humming sound to your exhaling breath.

Instruct participants to open their eyes. If time allows, lead a discussion by inviting group members to share their experiences with the group.

VARIATION

Lead a discussion by asking participants to suggest times in their day when it would be convenient for them to practice these exercises.

NOTES

I often do these exercises while lying in bed, relaxing in the bathtub, taking a break at my desk, or riding in a car or airplane. Some of them can also be done while driving, taking a walk, or waiting in line.

This activity seems to appeal especially to women. I believe that a stimulating facial massage will help to bring a more radiant natural glow to the complexion than any cosmetics.

The elderly also appreciate this technique a lot. Even those with physical limitations are usually able to reach their faces with their hands. I love to include this activity in my yoga classes for the elderly and then watch the radiant light in the eyes of my beautiful 80- to 96-year-old students.

World Travelers

*Move your body in creative ways using images
from worldwide locations and cultures.*

PURPOSES
To practice guided imagery.
To practice or promote creativity.
To teach relaxation techniques.

TIME
5–10 minutes.

MATERIALS
None.

INTRODUCTION

Guided imagery is a powerful technique for helping yourself
and others to direct the imagination for a specific purpose. In psy-
chotherapy, it is used to help clients find creative solutions to personal difficulties. In the healing arts, it often helps patients learn
ways to lower their blood pressure, strengthen their immune system, or shrink a tumor. In spiritual counseling, it may help indi-
viduals contact their inner source of strength and wisdom. Guided
imagery can be used very effectively as a relaxation technique. In the
following activity, imagery adds a new dimension to the enjoyment
of physical exercise.

PROCESS

Ask participants to move to the center of the room, spacing

themselves an arm's length from each other. Read aloud the following script, pausing briefly after each sentence:

Stand in a comfortable position
and let your arms relax at your sides.

Imagine that your long-lost, rich uncle
has recently returned from a trip around the world
and has decided to make it possible for you to take a
similar journey—
on one condition:
you must find some interesting ways to experience each new place
and appreciate the energy of the people who live there.

Your journey begins in Italy . . . in the wine country to the south.
Close your eyes and imagine the rolling hillsides covered with
vineyards.
After visiting there awhile you decide to help the peasants
stomp grapes.
Begin moving your feet
as though you were squeezing the juice from the thick sweet
grapes . . .
crushing the fruits with your heels . . . and your toes . . .
and the centers of your feet . . .
dancing around a little . . .
pressing your feet down into the layer of grapes beneath you . . .
working as fast as you can before the sun sets over the distant
hills . . .
and then you can rest.
(pause)

Your explorations take you on to the Middle East . . .
to Syria and Saudi Arabia.
Imagine hearing belly-dancing music . . .
watching exotic women in long flowing dresses and filmy
purple veils.

The women invite you to join them in their harem ritual . . .
you begin moving your hips in a figure eight-pattern . . .
swaying from side to side . . .
letting your pelvis move forward and back . . .
around and around . . .
as your shoulders and arms
begin to flow with the rhythms of ancient drums . . .
feeling the rhythm of your heartbeat . . .
and then rest.
(pause)

Now you are in Peru, high in the Andes
in a small village
where people have lived for centuries.
After watching the dancers for awhile,
you are invited to participate.
Bend your arms and let your elbows bounce against your ribs
as you shift your weight from one foot to the other . . .
back and forth . . .
joining in with the group . . .
making expressive, resonant sounds
to accompany your primal, powerful dance . . .
and then rest.
(pause)

Your next stop is in the heart of Africa.
From a distance, you hear the sound of drums,
Rhythmic and powerful, yet varied,
the sounds draw you closer and closer
until you discover the source,
a circle of drummers, beating their instruments,
communicating across the jungle in the ancient way.
You decide to join them, your body becoming your instrument.
Make fists and pound on your chest . . .

Mind-Body Magic

moving your hands up toward your shoulders . . .
and around your heart . . .
pound gently, quietly . . .
sending an intimate message of love . . .
then let the volume increase as you
pound vigorously, declaring to the world
the joy of living . . .
and then rest.
(pause)

Now you are in Brazil . . . in the middle of the rain forest.
Imagine the thick green jungle vines
the huge tropical blossoms of yellow . . .
and violet. . . and magenta . . .
Light rain is falling . . . gently and steadily.
Place your fingertips on top of your head . . .
letting the raindrops tap your scalp . . .
around the back of your head . . .
around your ears . . .
down the back of your neck . . .
across your shoulders . . .
up to the top of your head again.
The raindrops are falling harder now . . .
bouncing and splashing . . .
helping you feel awake and alive with their energy . . .
and then the rain begins to stop and you can rest.
(pause)

Let your imagination take you to Hawaii . . .
to your favorite beach
or to one which you can create in your mind.
Imagine yourself . . .
listening to the sound of the pounding surf . . .
hearing the cry of the seagulls . . .

letting yourself dive into a rolling wave . . .
beginning to move your arms . . .
swimming out to meet the breakers . . .
feeling the flow of the salt water over your body . . .
continuing to swim forward . . .
then turning over and doing the back crawl
feeling invigorated and strong.

As you swim back to shore
you realize that a puppy has run off with your towel . . .
and you are soaking wet.
On the beach now, begin shaking the water off your arms . . .
and fingers . . . off your right foot . . . and left foot . . .
and off both feet at once.
Now shake your whole body . . .
letting yourself be warmed and dried
by the tropical sun and sea breezes . . .
and then rest.
(pause)

Picture now your favorite vacation spot . . .
anywhere in the world . . .
and let yourself travel there . . .
noticing your surroundings . . .
aware of what season of the year it is . . .

what time of day or evening . . .
breathing in the energy of this place.

Now begin moving your body in some way that is related to
your special spot . . .
engaging in some activity that helps you feel alive and
energized . . .
or relaxed and peaceful . . .
taking a few moments to really enjoy where you are . . .
what you are doing . . . how you are feeling . . .

and then rest.
(pause)

And now you are home . . . back in your own neighborhood . . .
your own backyard . . . or porch . . . or balcony
on a beautiful sunny day . . .
reaching your arms up to the sky
full of thanks for your wonderful journey . . .
for the experiences you had . . . for your safe return home . . .
reaching up to the sun . . .
drawing its warmth down over your whole body . . .
feeling relaxed . . . and nurtured . . .
reaching up again. . . feeling balanced . . .
feeling whole . . . and at peace . . . with yourself . . .
and the world.

▓ Ask participants to open their eyes. Conclude the session by encouraging participants to share their experience with others in the group.

VARIATIONS

▓ Form small groups and ask participants to compare notes on their experience with guided imagery. Use the following questions to get them started:

  ▲ What were the most relaxing images for you?

  ▲ Where did you notice the most tension in your body?

  ▲ How could you incorporate these techniques in your day-to-day stress management?

▓ Solicit other relaxing images from the group and incorporate them into a group guided image.

Seven Up

Energize your body in seven ways
and find out "what's up?"

PURPOSES
To provide a quick stretch break in a long meeting.
To loosen up a group which is feeling tense.

TIME
2–3 minutes.

MATERIALS
None.

INTRODUCTION
Many of us sit for periods of time each day at our desks, in front of a computer, behind the wheel of a car, and around meeting tables. When fatigue and tension accumulate and need to be released, here is an easy stretch to lighten your energy and help you feel more relaxed and refreshed.

PROCESS
Ask participants to stand up and space themselves an arm's length from each other. Read aloud the following directions:

Wake UP: Pound your fists on your chest as you roar like Tarzan.

Reach UP: Stretch your arms up over your head (alternating right and left sides) as you pretend to be climbing a tree or a ladder.

Loosen UP: Shake and wiggle your whole body like a limp doll.

Lighten UP: Let your arms become wings or feathers as you let go and fly.

Open UP: Starting with your palms together in front of your chest, stretch your arms forward and out as you open up to the possibilities of the world around you.

Lift UP: Imagine drawing energy up from the earth as you reach down and then lift your hands up the front of your body and over your head.

Snuggle UP: Turn toward someone nearby you and give each other a warm hug.

Conclude the exercise by reminding participants of the importance of stretching throughout the day to relieve tension and renew their energy level.

NOTES

This is a favorite among college students and the elderly, especially the snuggle up part!

Bumper Cars and Ghosts

Interact with other people
in enlivening and relaxing ways.

PURPOSES
To provide a group icebreaker.
To introduce the benefits of playfulness for mind/body well-being.
To let go of tension in a group.

TIME
5–10 minutes.

MATERIALS
A cassette or CD player; cassette tape or CD of lively music (for bumper cars); cassette tape or CD of relaxing music (for ghosts).

PROCESS
Introduce the purpose of the exercise and read aloud the following instructions:

Find a place to stand where you have lots of room for yourself.
Use as much floor space as possible.

Cross your arms over your chest
and hold onto your shoulders with the opposite hands.

Close your eyes and picture an amusement park.
Picture the bumpers cars
in which people are laughing freely
and having a wonderful time crashing harmlessly into one another.

When the music starts, open your eyes
and begin to move around the room like bumper cars,
gently running into people,
touching hips and shoulders and backs.
Let yourself laugh and enjoy the gentle physical contact.
Make eye contact with the other people in the room.
Allow yourself to be silly and childlike.

(play the lively music for two minutes)

When the music stops,
return to your original place in the room.
Let your arms relax at your sides.
Close your eyes and rest for a few moments . . .
Let go of the active energy you have just experienced . . .
Allow yourself to become quiet and centered inside . . .
Imagine that you have become invisible . . .

When the quiet music starts,
open your eyes
and begin to move around the room like a ghost,
pretending that no one else is aware of your presence.
Avoid making eye contact with anyone.
Be very quiet
and feel as though you are floating from one place to another.

(play quiet music for two minutes)

  Reconvene the entire group and move on to the next part of
your agenda, riding the crest of energy in the room.

VARIATION

  After completing the activity, form small groups of 4–6 participants. Lead a discussion using the following questions:

   Which activity did you enjoy the most?

   Did you like the contrast between the two?

Was either activity difficult for you in any way?

Are there times and places in your life when you feel like you are moving around like a bumper car?

Have you ever experienced being in a crowd of ghosts?

NOTES

I had an amazing experience in the busy train station in Beijing where huge crowds of Chinese people seemed to "float around" each other without ever getting in each other's way. Watching thousands of people riding bicycles in the streets of Shanghai gave me a similar feeling. There was no "bumper car mentality" there at all. What can we learn from that culture about an alternative way to move during rush hour in Grand Central Station?

What a Character!

*Increase self-awareness through
role playing one of your personae.*

PURPOSES
To challenge tightly held roles in an intact group.
To help participants open up to different aspects of themselves.
To promote team building or problem solving activities.

TIME
15–20 minutes.

MATERIALS
A collection of hats (optional).

PROCESS
Introduce the topic and purpose of the exercise. Ask participants to think of a "character" that they have played within the last week. Give this character a name such as: Pushy Pat, Mournful Morgan, Busy Bud, Silly Sally, Winning Willie, Compassionate Clara, Accommodating Arthur, etc.

Ask group members to introduce themselves to others in the group as this character as they move around the room interacting with various people. Provide the following instructions to help them get started:

Act out the characteristics of this part of yourself.

Exaggerate the qualities that you are portraying.

- Talk to other people using this character's voice.

- Respond to others from this character's point of view.

- Notice how other people are responding.

- Allow yourself to "ham it up" and laugh at yourself.

- Interact with a variety of people and notice what feelings come up for you.

After 15 minutes, reconvene the entire group and ask participants to share any additional comments or insights they gained during this experience. Lead a closing discussion using the following questions:

- How did it feel to become this character?

- What did you learn about yourself?

- Was this fun for you?

- Was any part of it difficult?

- Who else do you know that would benefit from this activity?

NOTES

Sometimes I present my collection of hats from all over the world and encourage the participants to choose a hat to wear and then become the character that their hat suggests to them. We have a "get to know you party" in which we meet each other individually and then introduce ourselves to the whole group. In this case, I encourage people to become a character that is unfamiliar to them—someone from another culture, a different age group, the opposite sex, another time in history.

I have found this activity particularly effective with college students and young adults.

OPENING UP OUR CREATIVITY

The ten activities in this section offer opportunities to experience body-mind connections from the creative perspective. Creativity is closely related to imagination, which Albert Einstein called "more important than knowledge." Creativity also involves flexibility, risk taking, commitment, letting go, and a good sense of humor!

One effective technique for enhancing creativity is using affirmations or "telling the truth in advance." Another is the use of metaphors to give us a different slant on new connections between concepts and better relationships between people. The following activities will provide experiences for enhancing our creative process and helping us feel more fully alive. In the words of Joseph Campbell, we will be better able to "follow our bliss."

Free to Be Heard

Allow your voice to open you up
to creative self-expression.

PURPOSES
To prepare for creative activity or endeavor.
To demonstrate the kinesthetic component of creativity.
To allow sounds to promote freedom of expression.

TIME
10–15 minutes.

MATERIALS
Free to Be Heard worksheet; pens or pencils; easel pad and markers.

INTRODUCTION

Just as harsh sounds and industrial noises can be disturbing to our mental and physical well-being, pleasing music and sounds of nature can energize us, relax us, and bring us into a state of balance and wholeness. Music can affect our breathing, our heart rate, our blood pressure. It can promote healing, facilitate learning, and inspire devotion. Experiencing the vibrations of our own voices is a powerful way to stimulate our creativity and open up new channels of self-expression.

PROCESS

Explain the purpose of this exercise and give participants the following instructions:

- In a relaxed standing position, make the following vowel sounds in whatever way you wish:

  AH   AY   EE   I   O   OO

- Exaggerate each vowel sound by shaping your mouth very deliberately.

- Vary these sounds by making them higher/lower, louder/softer, longer/shorter.

- Add whatever body movements you wish to each sound.

- Now call out words and combinations of sounds such as:

Alleluia	Bravo	Zippity Doo Dah
Shalom	Hooray	Oo la la
Aloha	Yea	Aye yi yi
Amen	Wow	Ma Ma Ma Ma Ma

  or any other words or babbling sounds that may occur to you.

- Close your eyes and make as many nonsense noises as you wish, adding whatever body movements feel good to you. After several minutes, open your eyes and sit down.

Distribute the **Free to Be Heard** worksheet to participants to remain in this free, creative mode and ask them to complete it. Allow 5 minutes for this process.

If time allows, lead a closing discussion by asking participants to reflect on the insights they experienced during this activity.

VARIATIONS

After the worksheets are completed, form groups of 4–5 participants who have a common vowel in their first names. Ask them to share their experience and worksheet responses with each other.

After distributing the **Free to Be Heard** worksheet, list on the easel pad open-ended sentences related to a specific issue, topic, or problem of the group you are working with. Ask participants to use one of these phrases to begin their writing. For example:

If this conflict could speak, it would say . . .

I hope that next time . . .

This problem could be resolved by . . .

If I could change one thing, I would . . .

If I were in charge, I would . . .

If I could do it over again, I would . . .

NOTES

This is one of the best techniques I have ever found for freeing people's energy for creative writing.

©1997 Martha Belknap Whole Person Associates • 210 West Michigan • Duluth, MN 55802 • (800) 247-6789

Free to Be Heard

Choose one of the story-starter sentences or think of one on your own. Write whatever thoughts come to your mind.

What if . . .

Imagine that . . .

If I were free to . . .

As You B.R.E.A.T.H.E.

Use your breath to affirm
positive qualities related to creativity.

PURPOSES
To promote self-care, self-nurturing, or self-esteem.
To demonstrate an effective technique for getting unstuck and restoring a positive energy flow.
To prepare for a creative activity or problem-solving situation.

TIME
4–5 minutes.

MATERIALS
None.

INTRODUCTION
Our mental and emotional states are often reflected in the way we breathe. When we are feeling confused, tense, or scared our breath tends to become rapid and shallow. Conscious slow deep breathing brings more oxygen to our lungs and consequently to our brains for greater clarity, calmness, and energy. Breathing is one of the few physiological functions which is both automatic and also under our conscious control.

PROCESS
Introduce the exercise to participants and read aloud the following script:

Sit in a comfortable position with your feet flat on the floor.

Press the top of your head up toward the ceiling
so there is an easy flow of energy
from the top of your head to the base of your spine . . .

Close your eyes and become aware of your breathing . . .
Allow your incoming breath to be slow and deep.
Allow your outgoing breath be long and full.
As you breathe in, think to yourself, "I am expanding."
As you breathe out, think to yourself, "I am releasing."
I am expanding . . .
I am releasing. . . .
expanding . . .
releasing . . .

(pause for at least 8–10 breaths)

In the second part of this activity, ask participants to inhale when you read the words "Breathe in and" and exhale when you read each of the following phrases which begin with the letters of the word "Breathe:"

Inhale	**Exhale**
Breathe in and	B elieve in yourself
Breathe in and	R elease your tension
Breathe in and	E xpand your vision
Breathe in and	A cknowledge your strengths
Breathe in and	T rust your intuition
Breathe in and	H onor your individuality
Breathe in and	E njoy your creativity

Repeat this activity a few more times, encouraging participants to focus on the affirming phrases as they breathe.

Provide these instructions as you lead participants through the following breathing activity, using new words to help affirm other positive qualities related to creativity:

Inhale	Exhale
I breathe in	B alance
I breathe in	R elaxation
I breathe in	E nergy
I breathe in	A wareness
I breathe in	T ranquillity
I breathe in	H umor
I breathe in	E nthusiasm

Conclude the session by asking group members to think of some other words which have special meaning in their own creative process. Encourage them to use these affirming qualities as they use this exercise on their own.

VARIATIONS

Choose appropriate, energetic, affirming words that start with the letters of your own name. For example I use:

M indfulness		T rust	
A ppreciation		H umor	
R eceptivity		A wareness	

To build team spirit, brainstorm to come up with affirming words as acronyms for team or department names such as editorial:

E fficiency		R elevance	
D aring		I nitiative	
I deas		A ttention to detail	
T radition		L ove	
O rganization			

With young children, use posters of the letters and words to help fix them in their memory. Or give each child a different letter to hold up and a message word that begins with that letter. Then ask the children with letters to come up and spell the word for the whole class.

Magical Metaphors

Improve communication
of feelings by using metaphors.

PURPOSES
To demonstrate effective communication skills.
To teach relationship skills with couples or families.
To help resolve conflicts in the workplace.

TIME
10–15 minutes.

MATERIALS
Magical Metaphors worksheet; pens or pencils; easel pad and markers.

INTRODUCTION
Communication is an attempt to express our experience in common symbols. The more clearly we can describe our experiences and find common symbols, the higher the likelihood of our understanding one another. Metaphors can be extremely helpful in this process.

PROCESS
Explain the purpose of the exercise to participants. Distribute the **Magical Metaphors** worksheet and provide the following instructions:

Think of situations in which you want to communicate to

someone your feelings regarding something that person has done or said.

- Translate the feelings you have into images of nature or experiences you are both familiar with.

- State what you would like to have happen. Write down each of these responses under the appropriate heading at the top of each column on the worksheet. You will have 10 minutes for this process. I have listed some examples on the easel pad to help you get started.

Before the session begins, copy the following list onto an easel pad for participants to refer to as they think of their own examples.

Situation	**Metaphor**	**Request**
When you:	*I feel like:*	*I would like you to:*
snap at me harshly	a bolt of lightning has struck me	speak to me in a more sensitive way
agree to help me	the sun is shining in my heart	know how much I appreciate your kindness
ignore me	a cold wind is surrounding me	listen when I have something to tell you
appreciate me	I am snuggled up on Grandma's lap	know how much that means to me
forget to call for a long time	a plant that hasn't been watered	keep in touch more often
are attached to a rigid way of thinking	I am up dealing with a prickly cactus	be open to seeing things differently

When everyone has finished the worksheet, lead a closing discussion about the importance of clear communication. If time allows, ask participants if they would like to share their comments or insights on the topic.

VARIATIONS

Form groups of 4–5 participants and encourage group members to share their worksheet responses with each other. Encourage them to discuss the following questions:

- How could you use these metaphors in expressing feelings to people you know?

- Are there some people who would not respond well to this type of interaction?

Ask participants to use the **Magical Metaphors** worksheet to practice making metaphors for feeling-related experiences in different contexts.

NOTES

I have used this activity with a group of mothers and teenage daughters and also with groups of couples. Instead of writing their ideas on the worksheet, they sat face to face and spoke to each other. Below are examples of some of the comments which were shared:

Mother to her daughter: When you walk into the room, I often feel like an electric storm has shocked me. I would like your energy to be more like a gentle rain in the forest.

Daughter to her mother: When you keep watching everything I do, I feel like you are a cougar about to pounce on my back. I would like you to be a soft rabbit that I could cuddle in my arms.

Husband to his wife: When you keep repeating the same requests over and over, I feel like you are a drippy faucet which cannot be

Mind-Body Magic

turned off. I would like you to make your request clearly and then be patient.

Wife to her husband: When you are resistant to considering new ideas, I feel like I am experiencing a logjam in a river. I would like you to allow a flow of ideas between us so we can understand each other better.

   I have also found this technique to be useful with various age groups, including:

   Youngsters in conflict management training

   Adults in the workplace who need to set boundaries

   Older folks who may not be used to expressing their feelings

Magical Metaphors

Think of people you want to communicate with more clearly: a parent, your child, your partner/spouse, a coworker/neighbor, your boss, etc. Fill in the columns with your feelings in specific situations.

Situations	Metaphor	Request
When you . . .	*I feel like . . .*	*I would like you to . . .*

Mind–Body Magic

My Wildest Dreams!

*Combine goal-setting with
creative fantasy to enhance self-esteem.*

PURPOSES
To help clarify values.
To help set goals.
To promote imaginative thinking.

TIME
15–20 minutes.

MATERIALS
My Wildest Dreams worksheet; pens or pencils.

INTRODUCTION
Having a vision and putting it into words, both written and spoken, is an effective way to help our wildest dreams come true.

PROCESS
Introduce the purpose of the exercise to participants. Distribute the **My Wildest Dreams** worksheets and give instructions for completing the reflection process:

 Imagine yourself and your life at some time in the future.

 Use your creative imagination to fill in the blanks of all the sentences.

 Each sentence may represent a different aspect of yourself.

▲ Feel free to play with ideas in the realm of imagination as well as reality.

▨ Form groups of 4–5 participants and ask them to share their ideas and comments with each other. Have one person choose a sentence to read aloud and then have the others give their responses to the same sentence. Encourage people to expand on their ideas by asking questions such as:

▲ Why would that be important to you?

▲ Why would that be fun for you?

▲ Do you think you will ever have an experience like that?

▨ If time allows, conclude the session by reminding participants of the importance of having a vision and putting it into action to reach their goals.

VARIATION
▨ If you have extended time, combine this activity with **Cover Story** on page 93.

©1997 Martha Belknap Whole Person Associates • 210 West Michigan • Duluth, MN 55802 • (800) 247-6789

My Wildest Dreams!

I have been awarded an honorary degree from

in the field of

I have been invited by
on a nationwide tour in order to

There is a feature article about me in
for being chosen "
of the Year."

I have been invited to be a house guest at the home
of

The governor/president
has asked me to be a special consultant on

The government of   has
requested that I visit that country in order to

©1997 Martha Belknap Whole Person Associates • 210 West Michigan • Duluth, MN 55802 • (800) 247-6789

My Wildest Dreams! (continued)

▪ I have received a medal/prize/award for _____

_____

_____

▪ I have been invited by _____

to appear on national TV for _____

_____

▪ I have received recognition for my discovery/invention/

creation of _____

_____

▪ On my gravestone will appear these words:

_____

_____

_____

_____

Cover Story

Put personal dreams and fantasies into
written form to clarify and affirm them.

PURPOSES
To enhance self-esteem.
To help people know each other better.
To promote life-planning skills.

TIME
10–15 minutes.

MATERIALS
Cover Story worksheet; pens or pencils.

INTRODUCTION
Our images of the future affect our choices in the present and vice versa. Sometimes planting seeds in the form of suggestions to ourselves will have far reaching effects on future directions in our lives.

PROCESS
Solicit ideas from the group on accomplishments they are proud of, or would be proud of. Give lots of examples (e.g., learning another language, playing the "Moonlight Sonata," getting three kids through high school, running a marathon, raising a bowling average over 150, becoming a college president, learning to tie all the knots in the sailing manual, climbing Kilimanjaro, etc.). Tailor some examples to the group.

Ask participants to focus specifically on one accomplishment they would like to achieve in their lifetime. Ask them to imagine that in five to ten years they will be nationally recognized for an outstanding achievement that is of significance to them. Their picture will appear on the cover of a major magazine and a feature article will be written about them. Ask participants the following questions:

- What is the achievement?

- Is there an award involved?

- In what magazine does the article appear?

Distribute the **Cover Story** worksheet to participants and provide the following instructions:

- Write an article about yourself (in the third person) explaining what you have accomplished and why this is of importance.

- Use creative imagination combined with a clear focus upon a goal or dream which you would like to pursue. Mention the steps which led up to this achievement.

- When the article is finished, write a catchy headline that will intrigue readers and add some captions for accompanying photographs or illustrations.

When everyone has completed the worksheet, ask participants who are willing to share their worksheet responses. Lead a closing discussion on success based on the different ideas that were shared.

VARIATIONS

After writing your cover story, divide into small groups and share what you have written. Ask each other questions such as:

- How do you feel about receiving this recognition?

Is this story in line with your true aspirations or is it simply a wild fantasy that is fun to consider?

Post stories around the room for a break-time Hall of Fame gallery tour.

Read a few stories out loud to get a sense of the whole group. Then divide into small groups and have people read their own story out loud. Reading to an audience adds a powerful dimension to this self-affirmation.

There are those who view success as the arrival at a destination. Others see it as the enjoyment of the journey. Ask the group the following questions:

What is your concept of success: reaching a goal or the journey towards the goal?

Can you embrace both of these viewpoints at the same time?

NOTES

I have used this activity with the college students in my creativity classes at the University of Colorado. They agree that it is one of their most enjoyable assignments. Sometimes the recognition comes from the local PTA, and sometimes it is a Nobel prize. Sometimes the stories fall into the realm of humorous science fiction. You can imagine how much fun these papers are for me to read! I usually choose selected stories to read out loud in class without identifying the author and then see if the students can guess who wrote them.

©1997 Martha Belknap Whole Person Associates • 210 West Michigan • Duluth, MN 55802 • (800) 247-6789

Cover Story

Magazine:

Headline:

Article:

Captions for illustrations and photographs:

Mind-Body Magic

Limitation and Freedom

*Look at the energies in your life
that limit your freedom and the
energies that expand your freedom.*

PURPOSES
To facilitate resolutions for change.
To promote self-discovery.

TIME
10–15 minutes.

MATERIALS
Limitation and Freedom worksheet; pens or pencils; easel pad and markers.

INTRODUCTION
Just as a river needs a steady flow of energy to carry it onward, balanced human beings need a steady flow of energy to provide freedom from limitations and opportunities for change. Think of the words to the Serenity Prayer:

*Grant me the serenity to accept the things I cannot change,
the courage to change the things I can change,
and the wisdom to know the difference.*

At times, we stubbornly fight against a situation when, in fact, we would benefit more from serenity, acceptance, and courageous surrender. And there are also times when we resign ourselves to accepting "the way things are" when, in fact, we could seek the courage to make changes that would enhance our freedom.

PROCESS

▨ Introduce the topic and distribute the **Limitation and Freedom** worksheet. Provide the following instructions:

▲ Beginning with the heading "Mind," list the energies or qualities in your life which limit your freedom and those which expand your freedom. I've written some examples on the easel pad to give you ideas.

Before the session begins, copy the following list onto an easel pad for participants to refer to as they think of their own examples.

Mind
limitations: judgments, anxiety, addictive behaviors
freedom: clarity, creativity, receptivity

Body
limitations: fatigue, tension, compulsive eating
freedom: vibrant energy, strong immune system, spinal flexibility

Heart
limitations: resentments, guilt, anger
freedom: courage, compassion, forgiveness

Spirit
limitations: attachments, hypocrisy, separation
freedom: awareness, serenity, trust

▲ Continue completing the other three sections of the worksheet ("Body," "Heart," and "Spirit"). You will have 10 minutes for this process.

▨ After everyone has finished the worksheet, divide participants into small groups. Lead a closing discussion by asking participants to share what they have written including one of their limitations and one area of life in which they desire greater freedom.

VARIATIONS

Brainstorm with the group possible ways of overcoming personal limitations. For example: regular exercise, deep breathing, time alone in nature, nutritional awareness, journal writing.

Choose one specific change that you are ready, willing, and able to make this week. Write that idea on your worksheet in terms of an affirmation for the release of your limitation and an expansion to greater freedom in your life. For example: "In order to release tension from my body and enjoy more vibrant energy, I commit to talking a brisk walk for at least half an hour, at least three times a week."

Choose a partner in your group to be your "buddy," preferably someone who lives nearby. Share with that person the commitment you have written and exchange phone numbers. Agree to call regularly to encourage each other to stay committed to your chosen goals. You may want to agree to pursue your goals together if that is possible. For example, by taking a walk together or cooking a healthy meal for each other.

Limitations and Freedom

	Limitations	Freedom
Mind		
Body		
Heart		
Spirit		

Affirmation for change:

Rock, River, and Tree

Examine images in nature
as symbols of your life.

PURPOSES
To get a wider perspective on your life.
To promote self-exploration.
To focus and facilitate change.

TIME
10–15 minutes.

MATERIALS
Rock, River, and Tree worksheet; pens or pencils.

INTRODUCTION
We often use images of nature in our language to represent personal qualities or experiences. For example:

He is the Rock of Gibralter.
She has a rocky road ahead of her.
My life is bubbling along smoothly.
Their relationship is in the pits.
We are establishing roots for ourselves.

Let's explore these images in depth and discover how they can apply to our attitudes and behavior patterns.

PROCESS
Introduce the exercise and slowly read aloud the following script, pausing after each sentence:

Close your eyes and picture a large rock.
Notice what color and texture it is and where it is located.
Perhaps it is a rock you have seen somewhere in the world or it
could be a rock you are creating in your imagination.
Let this rock represent a firm foundation upon which you can
stand, a source of strength in your life.

What is there in your life which is steady and solid?
Do you have a good education, a satisfying job, a spiritual
practice, or a positive self-image which is a source of strength
for you?

Could your rock also represent an obstacle that is standing in
your way?
What is there in your life that gets in the way of accomplishing
your goals?
Do you have habits or relationships that restrict you? Attitudes
that get in your way?

For example: Do you overeat and say to yourself:
"I don't want to waste food so I'll clean my plate."
"I don't want to offend my hostess by refusing seconds."
"I paid a lot for this meal so I should eat it all."

After reading the above examples, instruct participants to open their eyes. Ask them to complete the top section of the worksheet, jotting down what there is in their life that can be represented by a rock.

After a few minutes, continue reading the script:

Close your eyes again and picture a river.
Let it be a real one you have enjoyed or one which you are
imagining.
Let the river represent the energy you are experiencing in your
life, the song you are singing.

What is flowing well for you right now?

*How is your health, your personal freedom, your creativity, your
sense of well-being?*
Does your river ever feel like it is raging?
Is it jumping its banks and flooding the surroundings?
Does it ever seem to be getting stagnant?

Direct group members to open their eyes and turn to their
worksheet again. Ask them to complete the middle section by writing down what there is in their life that can be represented by a river.

Continue reading aloud the script:

Close your eyes once more and picture a tree.
Is it a tree you are familiar with?
*Let this tree represent the changes that you are creating in
your life.*
In what ways are you growing and branching out?
*Are you developing more awareness, skills, trust, compassion,
peace?*
Are your goals rooted in fertile soil?
Is any part of you withering up?

Ask participants to open their eyes and invite them to complete
the bottom section of their worksheet by having them write down
what there is in their life that can be represented by a tree.

Explore the group's creative energies a little further by leading
participants in a closing discussion using these questions:

What else could you express about yourself and your life?

How can you draw strength from your rock?

How can you flow with your river?

How can you nourish your tree?

VARIATION

After completing the worksheet, form groups of 4–6 participants and encourage them to share their responses with each other. Use the following questions to stimulate discussion:

Are there some similarities within the group?

Did anyone in your group interpret these symbols in a way which had not occurred to you?

NOTES

This activity was inspired by a poem by Maya Angelou entitled "On the Pulse of Morning." It was read by the author at the inauguration of President Clinton in 1993. A recording of this poem is available from Random House AudioBooks. You may want to read the poem to the group as a warm-up or wrap-up.

Rock, River, and Tree

Rock

River

Tree

15 Ways to Clean the Kitchen Floor

Examine various approaches to situations in life that require change.

PURPOSES
To provide a humorous interlude that confronts our natural tendency to avoid change.
To illustrate the power of resistance.
To help understand some of the reasons for our behavior.

TIME
10–15 minutes.

MATERIALS
Seven Tendencies worksheet; pens or pencils.

PROCESS
Make five photocopies of the list of 15 Ways to Clean (or Not Clean) the Kitchen Floor on page 107.

▨ Imagine that your kitchen floor really needs to be cleaned. Select five participants to take turns dramatically reading the list of items. Ask them to not read the words in parentheses.

15 Ways to Clean (or Not Clean) the Kitchen Floor

1. "I see a little tomato sauce over here and some cereal over there. Which one did I spill first? Was it on Monday or Tuesday? What was happening at the time?" (overanalysis)

2. "I didn't spill that pickle juice. I never eat pickles. It must be someone else's fault." (shifting the blame)

3. What a terrible housekeeper I am! How disgusting to be so sloppy!" (self criticism)

4. "I'll take care of it some other time. I'd rather wait until I'm more in the mood." (procrastination)

5. "I'll just clean up the mess in the middle of the floor. No one will ever notice what's behind the refrigerator." (indifference)

1. "The floor isn't really that dirty after all. In fact, it looks just fine to me. No big deal." (denial)

2. "I'm part way through and that's all I'm going to do. Someone else can finish the rest." (shifting the responsibility)

3. "Well, maybe I'll just do a once over lightly cleaning job. Then at least I can say that I tried." (half-hearted attempt)

4. "I'm going to scrub and scrape and scour and I'll even use abrasives if I have to. I want this kitchen floor to sparkle!" (perfectionism)

5. "It's no use. No matter how hard I try, I can never get this floor clean. Why even bother?" (helplessness)

1. "Oh dear, I'd better clean it up. What would people think of me if they saw this messy floor?" (fear of disapproval)

2. "This damn floor! Why does it always have to get so dirty?" (displaced anger)

3. "Maybe if I just let it go a little longer, someone else will take care of it." (avoidance of responsibility)

4. "I'll do it because cleaning floors is part of my job. It's expected of me and I have no other choice." (resignation)

5. "I'll do it now—and when I'm finished I'll feel much better and the floor will be clean." (acceptance of responsibility)

Ask participants if they can think of any responses to a dirty floor that were not mentioned? Are the responses typical of anyone they know? If so, who and in what situations?

Ask participants to label the kinds of behavior they heard described. As necessary, prompt with requests for examples of:

- over-analysis

- denial

- blame

- procrastination

- perfectionism

- helplessness

- resignation

Explain to participants that these are all typical approaches we might take to any situation in life that requires change. Distribute the **Seven Tendencies** worksheets and invite people to identify instances when they occasionally or frequently use the behaviors listed in response to changes they should be making.

> *Give lots of examples of situations that might need attention (e.g., a report/analysis that needs to be written, a problem employee who needs confronting, a child not doing well in school, a volunteer group in conflict, etc.).*

VARIATIONS

Find a partner and discuss the thoughts you have about the following questions:

- Are any of these responses typical of you in other situations? If so, when and where?

- Are any of the responses appropriate at certain times and in certain places? If so, when and where?

- Which responses leads to the most effective results in your life?

- In what ways could you choose to "clean up your act?"

- How has this activity helped you to look at various approaches to situations that need attention?

Develop a list of responses that are more likely to create positive change. Figure out strategies for applying these responses to a specific situation in your life.

For workplace audiences, create a similar list appropriate to the setting: a dreaded project that needs to be completed, staff reviews, procedure changes, etc.

Seven Tendencies

1. Over-analysis

Situation

My response

2. Denial

Situation

My response

3. Procrastination

Situation

My response

4. Blame

Situation

My response

Mind-Body Magic

Seven Tendencies (continued)

5. Perfectionism
Situation _____

My response _____
_____
_____

6. Helplessness
Situation _____

My response _____
_____
_____

7. Resignation
Situation _____

My response _____
_____
_____

Keeping Creativity Alive

*Expand possibilities for enhancing
creativity by evaluating current choices
and exploring new strategies.*

PURPOSES
To expand our understanding of the creative process.
To enhance our awareness of our own creativity.
To explore new ways to become more creative.

TIME
10–15 minutes.

MATERIALS
Creativity Checklist worksheet; pens or pencils.

INTRODUCTION
The term creativity is typically used in a limited sense as it applies to art, music, theater, dance, poetry, etc. If we understand that creativity can refer to the ways we think, then everything we do can become a creative act including the way we dress, tell stories, arrange our belongings, manage our time, raise our children, and plan our vacations. According to Deepak Chopra, the characteristics of creative people include the ability to enjoy silence, to connect with nature, and to be childlike.

PROCESS
Introduce the creativity exercise with comments on creativity appropriate to the audience.

Distribute the **Creativity Checklist** worksheet to participants and invite people to assess their creativity.

After everyone has finished completing the worksheet, form groups of 4–6 participants and encourage them to share what they have observed about themselves.

Reconvene the entire group and ask participants to share any additional comments or insights they gained during this activity.

VARIATIONS

Give examples of situations when you have put one or two of these strategies to work for yourself. What was the outcome?

Encourage others to try some of the ideas which you like the best and which work well for you.

Creativity Checklist

Mark with an X the suggestions which you already follow. Mark with a ✓ other ideas which you agree with but have not put into practice yet. Add some original ideas of your own.

❑ Explore new areas of interest that really "turn you on."

❑ Trust your own intuition and sense of inner knowing.

❑ Seek out lively companions as inspiring role models.

❑ Find good teachers who are guides, not drivers.

❑ Become well informed from a variety of sources.

❑ Practice relaxation and stress release every day.

❑ Become more centered through meditation and quiet time.

❑ Challenge your mind with puzzles, brainteasers, and games.

❑ Seek opportunities for good comedy, laughter, play, and fun.

❑ Daydream, visualize, fantasize, pretend, and imagine.

❑ Keep notes of your inspirations, observations, and experiences.

❑ Get plenty of sound sleep; pay attention to your dreams.

❑ Stretch and exercise regularly; eat energizing food.

❑ Regard mistakes as natural stepping stones to discovery.

❑ Spend time close to nature, away from crowds and noise.

❑ Welcome the unexpected, listen to the outrageous, and consider the impossible!

❑

❑

❑

❑

©1997 Martha Belknap   Whole Person Associates   •   210 West Michigan   •   Duluth, MN 55802   •   (800) 247-6789

Mind-Body Magic

Real Estate Ad

*Develop self-awareness by
describing yourself in a creative way.*

PURPOSES
To get acquainted in small groups.
To enhance self-esteem.
To illustrate applications for the creative process.

TIME
10–15 minutes.

MATERIALS
Paper; pens or pencils.

PROCESS
Distribute paper and pencils to participants. Give them the following instructions:

   As though you were writing a real estate ad, describe yourself in detail—your appearance, interests, and lifestyle. Let your imagination run free! Include your physical features and memorable qualities, the closets and junk drawers of your personality, your hidden flaws, and your dreams and visions.

   This description of the author could be used as a model:

   Sturdy structure in peaceful mountain surroundings.
   Designed in 1937.
   High ceiling, trim lines, no bay windows.
   Long narrow staircases leading to the basement.

Beige exterior, gray roof, blue tinted windows.

Smoke-free and drug-free interior.

Occasional damages to the framework have been skillfully repaired.

Study area contains a variety of books, poetry, photographs, creative journals, maps of foreign countries, Spanish dictionaries, teaching credentials.

Eating area reserved for fresh fruits and vegetables, whole grains, very few animal products, no caffeine or alcohol.

Meditation and yoga space enjoyed daily.

After everyone has finished their description, instruct participants to use their own as an example to introduce themselves to others in the group.

VARIATION

Describe your dream house in such as way as to indicate what is important to you in your life. For example:

Living room contains cozy fireplace, piano, harp, good stereo system, no TV.

Storage area contains skis, bicycle, tennis racket, hiking boots.

Extra room contains sewing machine, shell collection, camera, loom.

NOTES

The idea for this activity came from an actual ad in the personal column of my local newspaper under "Women Seeking Men."

RELAXING INTO STILLNESS

The ten activities in this section offer opportunities to experience body/mind connections from the relaxation perspective. Silence and stillness are at the heart of all deep relaxation, personal reflection, expanded awareness, and spiritual growth.

Conscious breathing, guided imagery, and meditation are some of the ways to create a state of mindfulness and a closer communion with our inner selves. Let's learn to be grateful for the lessons of the past as well as courageous about the challenges of the future while remaining fully awake to the present moment.

These activities will help to quiet the overactive mind and relax the overactive body in order to bring more joy to the heart, more peace to the soul, and more freedom to our lives.

Be Still and Know

*Use your breath, simple words, and
drumbeats to create a quiet state of mind.*

PURPOSES

To prepare for meditation, guided imagery, or personal reflection.
To illustrate the dynamic of rhythm in well-being.
To introduce breathing as a basic and easy relaxation technique.

TIME

1–2 minutes.

MATERIALS

A small drum; a quiet area in which to sit comfortably in a chair or
on the floor.

PROCESS

Introduce the topic and purpose of the exercise to participants.
Ask them to find a comfortable sitting position and to close their
eyes. Provide the following instructions:

As you listen to the following words, breathe in on one line
and out on the next.

(inhale)	Breathe in	(drumbeat	drumbeat)
(exhale)	Let go	(drumbeat	drumbeat)
(inhale)	Be strong	(drumbeat	drumbeat)
(exhale)	And flow	(drumbeat	drumbeat)

(inhale)	Expand	(drumbeat	drumbeat)
(exhale)	Release	(drumbeat	drumbeat)
(inhale)	Be filled	(drumbeat	drumbeat)
(exhale)	With peace	(drumbeat	drumbeat)
(inhale)	Reach out	(drumbeat	drumbeat)
(exhale)	And grow	(drumbeat	drumbeat)
(inhale)	Be still	(drumbeat	drumbeat)
(exhale)	And know	(drumbeat	drumbeat)

Follow each line with two even beats on the drum. In this way each line will have four counts—two syllables and two drumbeats.

▒ Lead participants through this activity several times, letting the drumbeats get softer and softer.

VARIATIONS

▒ When you are finished with the activity, divide participants into pairs or small groups. Ask them to discuss their mind-body experience during this activity and any implications they see for their life.

▒ Try different pacings during the activity and ask participants to pay close attention to the mind-body effects of speeding up the rhythm and of stretching it out.

▒ When the activity is completed, ask participants to brainstorm a personal breathing mantra or verse they can use when they practice meditation or for times of personal reflection.

I Lift My Awareness

Focus attention inside
and increase awareness.

PURPOSES
To illustrate the power of breathing to calm the mind-body.
To prepare for creative or problem solving endeavors.
To heighten awareness of mind-body connections.

TIME
4–5 minutes.

MATERIALS
Duplicated copies of the verses to distribute later (optional).

PROCESS
░ Introduce the purpose of this activity and ask participants to find a relaxed sitting position. Read the following script, pausing briefly after each line:

Sit comfortably and close your eyes.
Check to be sure that your spine is straight.
Place your feet flat on the floor.
Let your hands relax in your lap.

Focus your attention between your eyebrows.
Become aware of your breathing.

Notice how your breath is flowing in and out very slowly.
Allow your breathing to become very quiet, very still.
Each time you inhale, feel yourself expanding.
Each time you exhale, feel yourself letting go.

As I read the following verses,
breathe in on one line and out on the next.

Lift your awareness	*(inhale)*
Breathe into your spine	*(exhale)*
Enter the silence	*(in)*
And stillness divine	*(out)*
Lower your shoulders	*(in)*
Let go of your chin	*(out)*
Soften your belly	*(in)*
And focus within	*(out)*
Deepen your breathing	*(in)*
And as you let go	*(out)*
Quiet your mind	*(in)*
So awareness can grow	*(out)*
Balance your body	*(in)*
So healing can flow	*(out)*
Open your heart	*(in)*
So compassion can grow	*(out)*
Lighten your spirit	*(in)*
So freedom can flow	*(out)*
Deepen your breathing	*(in)*
And as you release	*(out)*
Let your whole being	*(in)*
Experience peace	*(out)*
Lift your awareness	*(in)*
above the distractions of your mind	*(out)*
so that you may be free	*(in)*
to receive guidance	*(out)*
Lift your awareness	*(in)*
above the sensations of your body	*(out)*
so that you may be free	*(in)*
to experience healing	*(out)*

Lift your awareness	*(in)*
above the conflicts of your heart	*(out)*
so that you may be free	*(in)*
to express love	*(out)*
Lift your awareness	*(in)*
above the attachments of the world	*(out)*
so that you may be free	*(in)*
to radiate peace	*(out)*

Continue to sit quietly,
allowing your breath to be slow
your mind to be calm
your body to be balanced
your heart to be open
your spirit to be free
and your whole being to be peaceful

(pause for a few moments)

Let your breath become a little deeper
Become aware of the places where your body is touching the chair
Begin to stretch your fingers and hands, your toes and feet
Let your head roll gently from side to side
When you are ready, slowly open your eyes

Place your hands on your face and gently massage
your forehead and cheeks
Stretch in any way that feels good to you as you gradually
bring your attention back into the room

VARIATION

Ask participants to write verses of their own to guide themselves into inner awareness. Form small groups and encourage participants to share their ideas and experiences with each other.

Imagine That . . .

*Use imagination and positive affirmations
to encourage personal awareness and creative change.*

PURPOSES
To warm up to a planning process.
To explore self-esteem issues.
To use as a closing activity.

TIME
10–15 minutes.

MATERIALS
Imagine That . . . worksheets; pens and pencils; duplicated copies
of the script.

INTRODUCTION
░ Many athletes use visualizations and positive affirmations as an
integral part of their training. We know how much our mental state
affects the success of a golf swing, a tennis stroke, a free throw in
basketball, a dive, a run down a ski slope. How we see ourselves
performing, how we talk to ourselves, and how we maintain our
focused attention are of equal or perhaps more importance than the
amount of practice time or our skill level. Let's use the power of our
imaginations to enhance other areas of our lives.

PROCESS
░ Introduce the exercise and ask participants to find a comfortable sitting position. Read aloud the following script, pausing briefly
after each sentence:

Close your eyes . . .
Imagine that you have eliminated habits from the past that
interfere with your growth and happiness . . .

Imagine that you now approach challenges in your life
with expanded awareness and greater responsibility . . .

Imagine that you have the serenity and the courage to meet
obstacles and changes along the path of your unfoldment . . .

You perceive all experiences and relationships with the knowl-
edge that you are constantly being presented with lessons to be
learned . . .

You are taking charge of your life knowing that guidance is
always available to help you with your choices and decisions . . .

Imagine that you can expect success
and that you are willing to take responsibility for achieving it . . .

You are able to use the errors of the past
as valuable information for self-correction and change . . .

You are able to forgive yourself and others
for the unconscious choices and unloving decisions of the past . . .

Imagine that you are releasing
all obsessive mind chatter and compulsive behavior . . .

Imagine that you are letting go
of all limiting patterns and beliefs that no longer serve you . . .

You are on a steady path forward
on which you are restoring yourself to balance and wholeness . . .

You are able to trust that you and others are part of a larger
picture that you are learning to perceive and understand . . .

You are allowing your challenges to call forth the best in you
to help you live your life with wisdom, integrity, love, and joy!

When you are finished reading the script, ask participants to open their eyes. Distribute the **Imagine That . . .** worksheets and copies of the script. Invite participants to relate their experience during the activity with current issues in their lives.

After everyone has completed the worksheet, form groups of 4–6 people and encourage participants to share their responses to the activity and worksheet reflection.

Lead a brief closing discussion reminding participants of the power of our imagination and how it can affect all areas of our lives.

©1997 Martha Belknap   Whole Person Associates   •   210 West Michigan   •   Duluth, MN 55802   •   (800) 247-6789

Imagine That . . .

One habit from the past that interferes with my growth and happiness is:

One of the challenges in my life that requires more attention is:

One of the obstacles or changes I am experiencing right now is:

One of the lessons I am learning in my life these days is:

One way in which I am expecting success and taking responsibility to achieve it is:

Imagine That . . . (continued)

Check the following statements that are true for you.

❏ I am using my past errors as guides for self-correction.

❏ I am forgiving myself and others for unconscious choices and unloving decisions in the past.

❏ I am releasing obsessive thoughts and compulsive actions.

❏ I am letting go of limiting patterns and beliefs that no longer serve me.

❏ I trust that I am part of a larger picture that I am beginning to perceive.

❏ I am allowing life challenges to call forth the best in me.

One way in which I am restoring myself to balance and wholeness is:

_____

_____

_____

Something else I would like to add to these affirmations is:

_____

_____

_____

One of these affirmations that does not fit for me is:

_____

_____

_____

©1997 Martha Belknap   Whole Person Associates   •   210 West Michigan   •   Duluth, MN 55802   •   (800) 247-6789

Mind-Body Magic

Slow Down and Live

Use affirmations to slow down and
improve the quality of your life.

PURPOSES
To present an antidote to the stress of Type A behavior.
To stimulate self-exploration about time management and choice-making.
To explore lifestyle decisions.

TIME
10–15 minutes.

MATERIALS
Slow Down and Live worksheet; pens or pencils.

INTRODUCTION
   Somewhere on a continuum from the crawl of a prairie to the zoom of a metropolis there is a comfortable pace that suits our own lifestyle and personal taste. When we take time to pay attention to our internal rhythms, we become aware of the need to adjust our energies as we shift from one environment to another. Many of us are speeding through life like a racehorse when, in fact, we would be much happier if we were trotting along like a pony or simply grazing in a peaceful meadow.

PROCESS
   Introduce the topic and lead participants in a discussion of their attitudes about time. Begin by asking the following questions:

- Do you often feel rushed/hurried?

- Do you eat/talk/drive too fast?

- Do you wish you had more time to yourself?

- Do you tend to overschedule yourself?

- Do you allow yourself enough extra time for unexpected circumstances?

- In what ways could you learn to slow down?

- Do you ever practice slow deep breathing?

- How would slowing down help improve the quality of your life?

Instruct participants to close their eyes. Ask them to focus on the phrases you are going to read aloud at this time:

As I slow down I will learn to:
move more gracefully . . .
eat more consciously . . .
think more clearly . . .
learn more effectively . . .
laugh more joyfully . . .
listen more attentively . . .
respond more lovingly . . .
live more peacefully . . .

Ask participants to open their eyes. Lead a closing discussion by inviting participants to think about times and places where they have felt rushed and hurried and other times and places where they have felt slowed down and relaxed.

©1997 Martha Belknap   Whole Person Associates   •   210 West Michigan   •   Duluth, MN 55802   •   (800) 247-6789

Slow Down and Live

Think about the ways slowing down would help you improve the quality of your life. Use the following verbs as suggestions and complete these thoughts with your own words.

By slowing down I am able to:

speak more

express myself more

work more

teach more

understand more

love more

decide more

accept more

relax more

share more

serve more

appreciate more

pray more

meditate more

Continue, using other verbs and adverbs which have special meaning to you:

I would like to learn to:

_____ more

_____ more

_____ more

_____ more

_____ more

Rainbow Balloons

Use the colors of the rainbow
to enhance personal strengths.

PURPOSES
To revitalize after remaining seated during a presentation.
To develop a sense of wholeness and wellness.
To prepare for team building or problem solving.

TIME
5–10 minutes.

MATERIALS
A room with a carpeted floor or floor mats in the event that participants choose to lie down for the relaxation script.

PROCESS
▓ Introduce the purpose of the exercise to participants. Slowly read aloud the following verses:

Move into a comfortable relaxed position,
either sitting or lying down with your eyes closed.
Imagine that you and some friends are hiking in the hills.
It is late in the afternoon at the beginning of summer.
You are on the top of a ridge overlooking the valley below.

Find a place where you can sit down and rest for awhile.
Allow your eyes to gaze at the view in the distance
as you enter into stillness and silence.

Imagine that from over the edge of the ridge

*there floats up into view a large **red** balloon.*
It is being carried gently on the breeze and is drifting toward you.
You reach out your hand and take hold of the string.
As you draw the balloon closer to you,
the color red fills your awareness.
Red reminds you of your strength.
You are filled with healing energy and vitality.
As you breathe in you feel the red energy filling your body.
You know that you are strong.

*Soon an **orange** balloon appears.*
You reach out again and take hold of the string
while continuing to hold onto the red balloon.
As you draw the second balloon toward you,
the color orange fills your awareness.
Orange brings you thoughts of warmth and comfort.
Imagine sending warm feelings into your belly.
Fill your heart with warmth and compassion for others.
Let yourself experience the power of the color orange.

As you place both strings into one hand
*you notice a **yellow** balloon floating by.*
Reach out with your free hand and take hold of that string.
The color yellow is bright and clear.
Imagine bringing yellow energy into your mind
to help you think with clarity.
Let your thoughts expand as yellow fills your awareness.
You feel awake and alert.

*Next you see a **green** balloon.*
Again you draw that balloon into your colorful bouquet.
Green gives you a sense of new life and joy.
It is the color of springtime and new beginnings.
You feel balanced within as you breathe the color green.

Another balloon floats up from below.

This one is medium **blue**.
As you reach out for the string,
you are reminded of the vast expanse of the sky and the depth of the ocean.
Your thoughts expand with creative energy.
You become aware of the many ways in which you express yourself.
There is no limit to the ways that you can explore your own creativity.

The next balloon is a dark blue or **indigo**.
Reach out and add this balloon to your collection.
As you draw it in, you feel that this is a very special color.
It brings deep insight and wisdom.
Imagine that you can breathe this dark blue color into your awareness.
Feel a heightened sense of understanding and inner knowing.

You are now holding the strings of six balloons in one hand
Notice the array of colors.
They represent many aspects of the outer world
and many feelings inside.
There is one more color to be included.
As you gaze out toward the west,
let the **violet** of the sunset flood over you.
As you breathe into the stillness you feel embraced by serenity.
A violet balloon now floats within your reach.
Take hold of the string and know that your rainbow bouquet is now complete.
Violet helps you connect yourself with the source of all creation
and with a sense of peace which is beyond measure.
Take some time to enjoy the fullness and beauty of this moment.

You realize now that it is time for you and your friends
to continue your hike down the hillside.

You look at the collection of seven balloons in your hand
and you consider some possibilities.
Do you want to take the balloons with you?
Do you want to let them go one by one?
Do you want to release them all at once?
Do you want to keep one balloon as a special reminder to you?
Are you thinking about some other choices?
Take a moment to decide what you want to do.
Then carry out your plan.

When you are ready, begin following the pathway down the hillside.
The full moon is out and is lighting your way.
With each step begin to bring your awareness back to the present.
Become aware of where you are and what time it is.
Slowly open your eyes and bring your attention back into the room.

Ask group members to find three other people wearing the same color as they are. In these small groups encourage participants to share the experiences they had with their balloons.

Reconvene the entire group and ask participants to share any additional comments or insights they gained during the activity.

VARIATION
Combine breath and color using the following guided imagery. Breathe in on one line and out on the next.

I breathe in *red* and feel it flow	(inhale)
I'm filled with *health* as I let go	(exhale)
I breathe in *orange*, feel it flow	(inhale)
I'm filled with *warmth* as I let go	(exhale)
I breathe in *yellow*, feel it flow	(inhale)

I'm filled with *strength* as I let go   (exhale)
I breathe in *green* and feel it flow   (inhale)
I'm filled with *joy* as I let go   (exhale)
I breathe in *blue* and feel it flow   (inhale)
I'm filled with *peace* as I let go   (exhale)
I breathe in *indigo* and know   (inhale)
I'm filled with *light* as I let go   (exhale)
I breathe in *violet* and know   (inhale)
I'm One with All and I let go   (exhale)

Mind–Body Magic

Dream House

*Expand self-awareness through
the use of guided imagery.*

PURPOSES
To introduce participants to each other.
To provide an opportunity for self-assessment and self-understanding.

TIME
20–30 minutes.

MATERIALS
Dream House worksheet; assorted colored markers, crayons, and pens; writing paper and envelopes (optional); a carpeted floor or floor mats.

INTRODUCTION
Many of us have a strong interest in learning ways to bring ourselves and our lives into better balance—ways to integrate the body, mind, heart, and soul. Native peoples and folks who live close to nature seem to know much more about living in balance than those people who lead busy lives in modern cities. However, all of us can let our imaginations take us to a setting where we can examine our lives on four levels—the physical, mental, emotional, and spiritual.

PROCESS
Introduce the subject of the exercise and ask participants to find a comfortable relaxed position, either sitting or lying down, with their eyes closed. Slowly read aloud the following script:

*Imagine yourself walking across a beautiful meadow in the
mountains.*
Notice the time of day and the temperature of the air.
*Be aware of the season of the year and the various colors
around you.*
In the distance you see a small house with a front porch.
Smoke is coming out of the chimney.
As you get closer you notice a sign on the door.
*Your full name is written on the sign followed by the words
"Welcome—Please Come In—This is Your Home."*

As you enter you find yourself in a hallway with four doors.
One door is red with a sign that says "Hall of Health."
One door is yellow with a sign that says "Library of the Mind."
One door is green with a sign that says "Haven of the Heart."
*The last door which is blue has a sign that says "Garden of the
Spirit."*

*As you open the red door leading into the Hall of Health
you notice posters on the wall.*
*They are pictures of people you admire who are physically strong
and fit.*
Notice who they are—athletes, dancers, friends, family members.
*Take a moment to be aware of what you might learn from
each of these people about how to take care of yourself in a
healthy way.*
How can these people serve as good role models for you?

On another wall are two full length mirrors.
As you look into the first mirror, notice your physical appearance.
What are you aware of first?
What do you like about the way you look?
What would you like to change?
Next to the mirror is a button that reads "Desired Change."
As you press this button, the reflection in the mirror shows you

how you would appear if a desired change were to occur.
How do you feel as you look at this new image of yourself?

The second mirror is an x-ray picture of the way you
function inside.
Notice the condition of your spine, your internal organs, the flow
of energy in your body.
What else can you observe about yourself from this inside view?
What are you most aware of?
Next to that mirror is another button that reads "Desired
Change."
As you press this button, you see how your insides would
function if a desired change were to occur.
What feelings do you notice now as you look at this new x-ray?

Leave the Hall of Health and walk back into the hallway.
As you open the yellow door which leads into the Library of
the Mind you notice some maps and charts on the wall.
The shelves are full of books.
On the table there is some equipment—
perhaps a globe, a microscope, a telescope, a computer.
Notice what is there that could help you learn about the world
in a way that would be fun for you.
On another table are some art supplies and musical instruments,
some pens and blank journals, some craft tools.
Notice what is there that could help you express yourself
creatively in the ways you would enjoy the most.

Seated in a comfortable chair is a very special teacher—
either someone you have known in your life
or someone you have learned about.
Perhaps this teacher is from a different time in history
or a different part of the world.
Notice who this person is and how you feel.
This person hands you a book and says, "Here is a gift for you.

Now is just the right time in your life for you to be reading
this book."
Notice what the teacher gives you and how you feel about
receiving it.

Leave the Library of the Mind and walk out into the
hallway again.
As you open the yellow door leading to the Haven of the Heart,
notice the sense of comfort you feel as you enter this room.
There is a fire in the fireplace
and some of your favorite music can be heard in the background.
There is a soft carpet on the floor
and some comfortable pillows in a pile.
The lights are low.
In front of the fireplace is someone you care about very much.
Perhaps it is someone you have not seen since childhood,
a friend you have not heard from for awhile,
or someone who is very close to you now.
This person invites you to sit down
so you can spend some time together.
As you look into this person's face,
be aware of the warm feelings between you.
Spend some time listening to the conversation you have
and noticing the feelings you share.

When you are ready, say good-bye to your special friend
and prepare to leave this room.
Walk out into the hallway again.
Open the blue door which leads outside into the Garden of
the Spirit.
Notice what kind of trees are growing there.
What color are the flowers?
Take a moment to enjoy the fragrance in the air.
Notice the light shining through the branches of the trees onto a
clear pond.

Listen to the sound of the waterfall nearby.
Find a place to sit down where you can enjoy the view.
Feel the peace and reverence of this sacred garden.
Not far away is a large piece of marble into which is carved a
symbol.
You know there is some special significance here for you.
Take some time to reflect upon this symbol
and what it means in your life.
On the other side of the garden you see a path
leading through an archway.
On the arch is carved an inscription—
words which have a special message for you
at this time in your life.
Spend some time thinking about why this is so important to you.
Relax into the stillness and the silence
of this special place.

After a while, bring your attention back to this present time
and place.
Allow your breathing to become a little deeper.
Begin to wiggle your fingers and toes.
Let your head roll gently from side to side.
Feel your chest expand as you breathe in.
Become aware of the places
where your body is touching the chair or the floor.
When you are ready, slowly open your eyes
and become aware of the room and the people around you.

When participants have their eyes open and are sitting upright, distribute the **Dream House** worksheets and invite people to extend their inner journey. Provide the following instructions:

On the worksheet, the words "Body," "Mind," "Heart," and "Spirit" are printed. Using colored markers, crayons, or pens, draw or write under each word something to represent what you experienced in each area of your house.

At the bottom of the worksheet, write a reminder to yourself of something to be more aware of in each area of your life. Make note of the people, the feelings, the gifts, the messages that were part of your imagery experience.

When everyone has finished completing the worksheet, form groups of 4–6 participants and invite them to share what they have drawn and written.

NOTES

I have used this activity with "at risk" teenagers. They are often able to express a lot of insights about themselves and about the changes they need to make in order to bring their lives more into balance. Sometimes I ask them to write a letter to themselves about these ideas, including a promise to themselves of some specific change they want to commit to. They sign the letter, put it into a self-addressed envelope, seal it, and give it to me to mail to them in a month—or six months. I have received many phone calls and postcards from these young people telling me how meaningful it was to receive the letters they had written and often forgotten about.

©1997 Martha Belknap Whole Person Associates • 210 West Michigan • Duluth, MN 55802 • (800) 247-6789

Dream House

Using colored markers, crayons, or pens, draw or write something to represent what you experienced in each area of your house.

Body   **Mind**

Heart   **Spirit**

Write a reminder to yourself of something to be more aware of in each area of your life. Make note of the people, the feelings, the gifts, and the messages that were part of your imagery experience.

_____

_____

_____

_____

Mind-Body Magic

Cruising Down the River

*Expand personal awareness using an imaginary trip
down a river as a metaphor for the journey of life.*

PURPOSES
To demonstrate assertiveness skills or personal empowerment.
To promote personal growth and development.
To enhance self-esteem.

TIME
10–15 minutes.

MATERIALS
Paper; pens or pencils; a carpeted room or floor mats.

PROCESS
In this exercise, participants will be asked to lie on the floor. Make sure you choose a carpeted room or provide floor mats. Ask participants to space themselves so they have plenty of room to find a comfortable position for this guided imagery exercise. Read aloud the following script, pausing briefly after each sentence:

Lie down on the floor and close your eyes.
Imagine your favorite river on a warm summer afternoon.
You are moving slowly downstream, fully aware of everything around you.

Focus your attention on your boat . . .
Perhaps it is a canoe, a raft, a kayak, a sailboat . . .
It represents your whole life at this moment,
your past, your present, and your future.

Focus your attention on your paddle, oar, rudder,
or whatever you are using to steer your vessel . . .
This is the way you direct the course of your life.
It represents your conscious choices, your use of creative thinking,
your ways of taking control and responsibility.

Focus your attention on the current of the river . . .
This is the natural flow of life through which you are always
moving without any conscious effort on your part.

Focus your attention on the reeds growing in the water . . .
They are firmly rooted to the bottom of the river
but are free to shift spontaneously with the changing current.
If they resist the flow they may break in half.
They represent the ways you allow yourself to move freely and
gracefully with the flow of life.

Focus your attention on the leaves floating in the water beside
your boat . . .
These are the imaginative thoughts in your own stream of
consciousness.
As you allow them to go where they want to,
without pushing them or stopping them,
they will naturally find their own channels of creative expression.

Focus your attention on the banks of the river . . .
These are the boundaries which give structure to life and direc-
tion to the flow of water.
Without these banks, the water would wander aimlessly and end
up in a stagnant bog.
The banks are the traditions, the teachings, the laws by which
you live.

Focus your attention on the wind . . .
This is the external power guiding you along on your journey.
If you try to fight against it, you may capsize.

If you allow yourself to make use of its energy,
your journey will most likely be safer and more direct.

Focus your attention on the boulders in front of you . . .
No one is there to move them aside for you.
You must learn how to avoid these obstacles by preparing ahead.
How do you use the power of your mind and body
to prevent yourself from getting hung up on these rocks?

Focus your attention on the shallow water . . .
You can see right through it. It has no depth.
It is of no use in propelling your boat.
Are there some shallow areas of your life which have no sub-
stance to them, no importance to you on your journey?

Focus your attention on the rapids . . .
You may feel some growing tension within you as you approach
the whitewater ahead.
You know these are difficulties for you to face head on,
challenges for you to meet and conquer.
How can you prepare yourself to run these rapids with courage
and confidence?

Focus your attention now on a lagoon . . .
Off to the side of the river there is a quiet resting place away
from the mainstream.
It is a spot where you can relax, meditate, and perhaps take time
to revise your itinerary.
It is also a good place to soak in the sunshine.

Focus your attention on the birds overhead . . .
They represent the freedom with which you can soar as you
begin to realize your potential,
as you become aware of who you are and how high you can fly.

Notice the storm in the distance . . .
You may need to take refuge for awhile and gather your strength
together.

*You may need to ask for extra protection or extra energy to
sustain you through a crisis.*
*How do you tap into your own source of strength and power
when you sense a storm is ahead?*

Focus your attention back on the sun . . .
*There is a constant and abundant source of light, warmth, and
energy which comes to you unasked for.*
*Are you always aware that this supply of energy is available
to you?*

Focus your attention on the clouds . . .
*These are the defenses you create to shield yourself from the
source of light and from other people's love.*
As you learn to push these clouds aside,
*you have a clearer view of life and a more meaningful connection
with others.*

Focus now on the sky overhead . . .
*Look up at the heavens and see a wider vision of possibilities,
an unbounded expansion of your potential.*
*Allow yourself to be lifted up to another state of awareness,
another state of being where your spirit is free to soar.*

*Gradually bring your awareness back to your own boat,
to your own life . . .*

When you are finished reading the guided imagery script, ask
participants to open their eyes and return to a sitting position. Form
small groups and ask participants to discuss their response to the
images in the script.

Reconvene the entire group and conclude the session by asking
for any additional comments or reflections the group would like to
share at this time.

VARIATIONS

▪ Distribute paper to participants and ask them to draw a diagram or picture of their life river right now and into the future. Then re-pose each question posed in the sections of the script, asking people to respond with a written or graphic representation on their drawings.

▪ Have participants close their eyes and listen to the following poem as you read it aloud very slowly:

Imagine a muddy river trickling aimlessly,
bogged down by weeds and snags, stagnant with debris, wandering nowhere,
bored with its own journey.

Imagine a dammed up river,
stuck behind a pile of heavy logs, unable to flow forward,
holding back its power,
about ready to spill over, scared of its own journey.

Imagine a river struggling to flow uphill, wasting all its energy,
battling against its nature, worn out by its efforts,
unwilling to redirect itself, frustrated by its own journey.

Imagine a raging river,
teeming with whirlpools,
plunging impatiently onward, crashing into boulders,
swept along by its own intensity, lost on its own journey.

Imagine a steady river,
following a clear course,
bubbling through the rapids, resting in quiet lagoons,
prepared for surprising waterfalls, directing its own journey.

Become a Star!

*Use a mnemonic device to remind yourself
to release tension from your body
as you focus your attention inside.*

PURPOSES
To teach relaxation skills.
To reinforce the pattern of relaxation breaks during the day.
To demonstrate the use of mnemonic devices as an aid to learning.

TIME
1–2 minutes.

MATERIALS
None.

INTRODUCTION
A mnemonic is a memory device which triggers the recall of information or reminds us to do something. Most of us have mnemonics which we learned in childhood to help us remember specific facts in school. For example: the word "homes" contains the first letters of the five Great Lakes. The following mnemonic will help us remember to smile and breathe. When practiced regularly it will aid us in establishing relaxation as a consistent quality in our daily lives.

PROCESS
Introduce the purpose of the exercise and provide the following instructions to participants:

Sit comfortably with your eyes closed.
Become aware of slow, deep breathing.

In your mind's eye picture a star and see the word
STAR written in front of you.
Using the four letters in the word S–T–A–R,
remind yourself to release tension from various parts of your
body.

S   *Smile*
T   *Take a deep breath (inhale)*
A   *And*
R   *Relax your eyes   (exhale)*

With relaxed eyes, begin to focus inside
and feel yourself radiating LIGHT . . .

Smile . . .
Take a deep breath . . .
And
Relax your jaw . . .

With a relaxed jaw, smile inwardly
and feel yourself radiating JOY . . .

Smile . . .
Take a deep breath . . .
And
Relax your shoulders . . .

With relaxed shoulders, expand your heart,
and feel yourself radiating LOVE . . .

Smile . . .
Take a deep breath . . .
And
Relax your belly . . .

With a relaxed belly, find your own center
and feel yourself radiating PEACE . . .

NOTES

My favorite times to practice this activity are:

upon awakening in the morning

before meditating

before eating a meal

when I am "on hold" on the telephone

before starting to drive a car

before going to sleep

and anytime during the day when I need to release tension from any part of my body

Joan Halifax, the noted anthropologist and author, tells the story of a particularly stressful day when she arrived at the Denver airport feeling rushed, not sure she would get to her plane on time. An elderly skycap looked at her kindly and said, "Ma'am, just remember to breathe and smile"—a message she had been hearing from Buddhist monks for years. Sometimes our best lessons come to us from teachers who appear in our lives wearing interesting disguises.

VARIATIONS

With the group (or in small groups) brainstorm situations in which the STAR relaxation sequence would be useful.

In small groups compose additional mnemonic devices to stimulate relaxation sequences. For example, with teenagers, use the music or movie star metaphor for your STAR sequence.

In the business setting, solicit examples of situations that make people uptight. Then teach the technique and ask teams to make up their own acronym to use. Teams could also develop a code word to use with each other to signal the need to calm down.

Sounds of Silence

Use your imagination to enjoy
the sounds of nature and of silence.

PURPOSES
To demonstrate the power of sensory experience in shaping mood
and attitude.
To use as a centering activity.
To stimulate creativity.

TIME
5–10 minutes.

MATERIALS
None.

PROCESS
Introduce the exercise and read aloud the following script,
pausing briefly after each sentence:

Assume a comfortable sitting position with your spine straight
and your hands resting in your lap.

Close your eyes and focus your attention on your breath.
Listen to the quiet sound of air as you inhale . . . exhale . . .
inhale . . . exhale . . .
Allow your breath to become so quiet that you are not aware of
any sound at all.

Imagine that you have been walking through the forest.
In the distance there is a bubbling brook.

As you get closer, the sound becomes clearer.
You can hear the water tumbling over the rocks creating tiny waterfalls.
Take a moment to listen to this joyful sound.

(long pause)

The river flows onward toward the sea.
In the distance you hear the pounding of the ocean.
As you get closer, the sound of the surf becomes louder.
The breakers are crashing along the rocky coast.
Let your breath move into tempo with the flow of the waves.
Take a moment to listen to these powerful ocean sounds.

(long pause)

You are in a meadow in the springtime.
The sun is beginning to go down and the insects are singing.
The crickets are chirping . . . the bees are buzzing . . .
some other creatures you can't identify are tuning up their tiny instruments.
Take a moment to listen to the meadow orchestra rehearsing.

(long pause)

As the music begins to fade, you hear the sound of tinkling bells.
Perhaps they belong to some tiny elves and leprechauns.
The sound is very light and gentle, barely audible.
Listen carefully as the magical tones drift into your awareness.

(long pause)

The sun disappears behind a large storm cloud.
You feel a few drops of rain.
Nearby is a large shelter with a strong tin roof.
You run over and duck inside seeking protection from the rain and wind.

You sit down on an old log and rest for awhile.
Listen to the sound of the raindrops on the roof.

They are falling faster . . . faster . . . and seem to be bouncing as they land.
Is there a rhythm to the rain? Is it changing?
Can you hear the whistling wind as well?
And the booming thunder in the distance?

(long pause)

The storm is over now. A silver mist is rolling over the meadow.
You are entering an enchanted land of unicorns and angelic beings.
In the distance a flute begins to play. Listen to the clear notes of the simple melody.
Feel the vibrations reaching your ears . . . and your heart.

(long pause)

As the flute begins to fade away, a harp begins its song.
A few notes at a time . . . a long pause . . . a few more notes . . . another pause . . .
the music is coming to you from very far away.
Listen . . .
Who do you think is playing? Who is singing?

(long pause)

The setting sun is sinking behind the distant hills.
The air is still warm and you have a blanket to spread out on the grass.
As you lie down, look up at the twilight sky.
The heavens are coming alive with sound.
The vibrations begin with a slow quiet hum . . .
and soon you hear the orchestra of creation . . .
a cosmic symphony echoing harmony throughout the universe.
Listen . . .

(very long pause)

Enter the silence . . .

Be quiet and know . . .
Deepen your breathing . . .
And follow the flow . . .
Lift your awareness . . .
Be still and release . . .
Listen to nature . . .
Experience peace . . .

(another long pause)

Become aware of your breathing as the music gets softer . . . and
softer . . . and softer.
Bring your awareness back to your physical being
and notice where your body is making contact with the floor.

Begin to move slowly . . .
wiggle your fingers and hands . . . your toes and feet . . .
let your head roll gently from side to side.
Deepen your breathing as you become more aware of this
moment in space.

Gradually, when you are ready,
open your eyes and become aware of your present surroundings.
Look around and tune into the energy in the room.
Notice what you are feeling inside.

Conclude the session by asking participants to turn to someone who is nearby and quietly share with them what they experienced during this activity.

VARIATION

Invite participants to sit back to back with a partner and practice sensory awareness. Provide the following instructions:

Select one person to start. The person selected will spend three minutes tuning in to their sensations, and as they notice them, they will describe them to their partner. Use the format, I am aware of . . .

The second partner listens only and supplies the support of a strong back for the first partner to lean against. Remind participants to pay attention to all five senses. Switch roles after 3 minutes.

When the second person is finished, turn face to face and talk about what you experienced.

Reconvene the entire group and ask participants to share any additional comments or insights they gained during this activity.

Am I Singing My Song?

Relax by reliving some moments of your past through the use of poetry and auditory memories.

PURPOSES

To promote relaxation.

To help explore personal empowerment.

To clarify values and explore life purpose.

TIME

5–10 minutes.

MATERIALS

Copies of the following poem (optional).

PROCESS

Explain the purpose of the exercise. Ask participants to find a comfortable sitting position and close their eyes. Read aloud the following poem:

Am I singing the song that I came here to sing?
Am I bringing to earth all the joy I can bring?
Am I dancing to music composed from above,
Vibrations of harmony, beauty and love?

Am I keeping my life in a natural key
So that I may become what I came here to be?
As I think, so I am; as I'm living I find
That my life has a tempo in tune with my mind.

Am I feeling those rhythms within and afar,

Directing my heartbeat—or guiding a star?
Am I hearing the symphony nature plays?
Composed in eternal and infinite ways?
Am I chanting the song that accompanies birth
of the wonder and joy of existence on earth!

Now with your eyes still closed . . .
imagine being in a large meadow on a warm summer s day . . .
a meadow you are familiar with . . . or one which you are
creating in your mind . . .
You are listening to the sounds of the birds . . .
hearing them singing to each other . . . noticing their melodies . . .
their harmonies . . .
their warbling . . . their chirping . . . their gentle cooing . . .
listening to their choir . . .

Imagine now that you are sitting in a very comfortable chair
with a happy baby in your arms . . .
listening to the sound of gentle breathing . . . the babbling . . .
the joyful laughter . . .
You begin humming a quiet lullaby and the baby is listening . . .
smiling with contentment, enchanted with the moment . . .

You have wandered into a huge stone cathedral with a vaulted
ceiling . . .
the choir boys are ready to begin practicing . . .
their pure voices are filling the air with angelic vibrations . . .
the boys are singing unaccompanied . . . in unison . . .
their tones are resonating with clarity and beauty . . .
you feel your spirit being uplifted by the magic of their melody . . .
and the simplicity of their sound . . .

Let yourself hear some other music which has a very special
meaning to you . . .
a melody from childhood perhaps . . . a love song . . . one of
your favorite dance tunes . . .

allowing the theme to run quietly through your brain . . .
bringing back a memory reminding you of a treasured time . . .
a particular place . . . a special feeling . . .

(long pause)

Now begin quietly humming to yourself . . .
allowing the notes to come to you gently and easily . . .
letting yourself tune into the rhythm . . . and the melody . . .
as you continue to hum softly to yourself . . .
allowing the tones to float into your awareness . . .
disregarding the other people in the room . . .
fully enchanted by your own music . . .
and your own special song . . .

VARIATION

Instruct participants to find two or three partners and encourage them to share what they experienced during this activity with each other. Use the following questions to get started:

- What song did you begin humming?

- Was it a song you recognize?

- Did you make it up?

- Are there words to the song?

- Is there some significance of this song in your life right now?

NOTES

Although generally I like to have background music to accompany guided imagery activities, in this experience I prefer quiet. In this way the listeners are freer to hear their own inner sounds and silences.

If the participants have copies of the poem that was read earlier, they may want to discuss the significance of "singing the song that I came here to sing" as it relates to finding your life purpose and following it.

⬜ Ask participants to write appropriate lyrics to the tune of their song.

Recommended reading

Belknap, Martha. *Taming Your Dragons* and *Taming More Dragons*. Boulder, Colorado, 1994.

Chopra, Deepak, M.D. *Quantum Healing*. Bantam Books, New York, 1989.

Douillard, John. *Body, Mind, and Sport*. Crown Trade Paperbacks, New York, 1994.

Fairfax, Joan. *The Fruitful Darkness*. Harper, San Francisco, 1993.

Huang, Chungliang Al. *Tai Ji*. Celestial Arts, Berkeley, 1989.

Naparstek, Belleruth. *Staying Well with Guided Imagery*. Warner Books, New York, 1994.

Northrup, Christiane, M.D. *Women's Bodies, Women's Wisdom*. Bantam Books, New York, 1994.

Paramahansa Yogananda. *Autobiography of a Yogi*. Self-Realization Fellowship, Los Angeles, 1994.

Redfield, James. *The Celestine Prophecy*. Satori Publishing, Hoover, Alabama, 1993.

Ryan, Regina Sara and John Travis, M.D. *Wellness: Small Changes You Can Use to Make a Big Difference*. Ten Speed Press, Berkeley, 1991.

Siegel, Bernie S., M.D. *Love, Medicine & Miracles*. Harper and Row, New York, 1986.

Swami Satchitananda. *Integral Yoga Hatha*. Integral Yoga Publications, Buckingham, Virginia 1995.

Thich Nhat Hanh. *The Miracle of Mindfulness*. Beacon Press, Boston, 1992.

Weil, Andrew, M.D. *Natural Health, Natural Medicine*. Houghton Mifflin, Boston, 1995.

OTHER WHOLE PERSON RESOURCES

INSTANT ICEBREAKERS
50 Powerful Catalysts for Group Interaction and High-Impact Learning

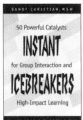

Sandy Stewart Christian, MSW
and Nancy Loving Tubesing, EdD, Editors

Introduce the subject at hand—and introduce participants to each other with these proven strategies that apply to all kinds of audiences and appeal to many learning styles.

Step-by-step instructions and dazzling graphics on the worksheets make any presentation a breeze.

❑ **Instant Icebreakers / $24.95**
❑ **Instant Icebreakers Worksheet Masters / $9.95**

PLAYFUL ACTIVITIES FOR POWERFUL PRESENTATIONS

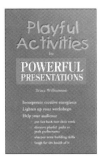

Bruce Williamson

Spice up presentations with healthy laughter. The 40 creative energizers in **Playful Activities for Powerful Presentations** will enhance learning, stimulate communication, promote teamwork, and reduce resistance to group interaction.

This potent but light-hearted resource will make presentations on any topic more powerful and productive.

❑ **Playful Activities for Powerful Presentations / $21.95**

MUSIC ONLY AUDIOTAPES AND CD

No relaxation program would be complete without relaxing melodies to play as background for a prepared script or to enjoy favorite techniques on your own. The melodic, solo guitar music of Steven Eckels is the perfect accompaniment for meditation, prayer, t'ai chi, yoga, journaling, periods of creativity, or relaxation. These "musical prayers for healing" will calm your body, mind, and spirit.

Audiotapes—$11.95 each

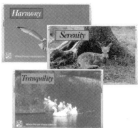

❑ **Harmony /** Waves of Light 30:00, Rising Mist 10:00, Frankincense 10:00, Angelica 10:00
❑ **Serenity /** Radiance 20:00, Quiescence 10:00, Evanescence 10:00
❑ **Tranquility /** Awakening 20:00, Repose 20:00

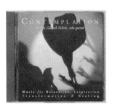

CD—$15.95 each

❑ **Contemplation /** Mystical Medition 31:33, Musical Mantras 31:05

**Call 1-800-247-6789 to receive a catalog
or to place an order. Or visit our website at
http://www.wholeperson.com/~books**

RELAXATION RESOURCES

Many trainers and workshop leaders have discovered the benefits of relaxation and visualization in healing the body, mind, and spirit.

30 SCRIPTS FOR RELAXATION, IMAGERY, AND INNER HEALING, VOLUMES 1 & 2
Julie Lusk

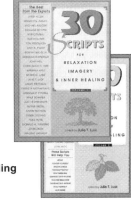

The relaxation scripts, creative visualizations, and guided meditations in these volumes were created by experts in the field of guided imagery. Julie Lusk collected their best and most effective scripts to help novices get started and experienced leaders expand their repertoire. Both volumes include information on how to use the scripts, suggestions for tailoring them to specific needs and audiences, and information on how to successfully incorporate guided imagery into existing programs.

❑ **30 Scripts for Relaxation, Imagery, and Inner Healing Volumes 1 & 2 / $21.95 each**

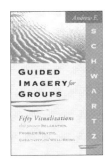

GUIDED IMAGERY FOR GROUPS
Andrew Schwartz

Ideal for courses, workshops, team building, and personal stress management, this comprehensive resource includes scripts for 50 thematic visualizations that promote calming, centering, creativity, congruence, clarity, coping, and connectedness. Detailed instructions for using relaxation techniques and guided images in group settings allow educators at all levels, in any setting, to help people tap into the healing and creative powers of imagery.

❑ **Guided Imagery for Groups / $24.95**

INQUIRE WITHIN
Andrew Schwartz

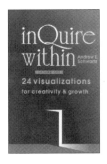

Use visualization to help people make positive changes in their lives. The 24 visualization experiences in **Inquire Within** will help participants enhance their creativity, heal inner pain, learn to relax, and deal with conflict. Each visualization includes questions at the end of the process that encourage deeper reflection and a better understanding of the exercise and the response it evokes.

❑ **Inquire Within / $21.95**

Call 1-800-247-6789 to receive a catalog or to place an order. Or visit our website at http://www.wholeperson.com/~books

WHOLE PERSON PRODUCTS

Stress & Wellness Series
* Structured Exercises in Stress Management Volumes 1–5 (softcover) .. each $29.95
  Structured Exercises in Stress Management Volumes 1–5 (loose-leaf) . each $54.95
* Structured Exercises in Wellness Promotion Volumes 1–5 (softcover) .. each $29.95
  Structured Exercises in Wellness Promotion Volumes 1–5 (loose-leaf) . each $54.95
  Stress & Wellness Reference Guide (index to series) $29.95

Tools for Working with Groups
* Working with Women's Groups Volumes 1 & 2 .... each $24.95
* Working with Men's Groups $24.95
* Working with Groups from Dysfunctional Families $24.95
* Working with Groups on Spiritual Themes $24.95
* Celebrating Diversity ....*................................... $24.95
* Bridging the Gender Gap $24.95
* Confronting Sexual Harassment $24.95
* Working with Groups to Explore Food & Body Connections $24.95
* Working with Groups to Overcome Panic, Anxiety, & Phobias $24.95
* Working with Groups to Explore Family Issues $24.95
* Working with Groups: Creative Planning for the Second Half of Life $24.95

Working with Young People
* Wellness Activities for Youth Volumes 1 & 2 .... each $21.95
  What Do You Do with a Child Like This? $15.95

Trainers Resources
  Playful Activities for Powerful Presentations $21.95
  30 Scripts for Relaxation, Imagery, & Inner Healing Volumes 1 & 2 .... each $21.95
  Inquire Within (imagery / meditation) $21.95
  Guided Imagery for Groups $24.95
  Mind-Body Wellness: An Annotated Bibliography $29.95
* Mind-Body Magic $24.95
* Instant Icebreakers $24.95

* Companion Worksheet Masters are available for all books marked with a *
  Worksheet Masters .... each volume $9.95

Self-Help Books
  Kicking Your Stress Habits $15.95
  Seeking Your Healthy Balance $15.95
  Overcoming Panic, Anxiety, & Phobias $12.95
  Sleep Secrets $12.95
  Don't Get Mad, Get Funny $12.95

Video Resources
  Making Healthy Choices Series (6 videos, Leader & Skill Building Guides) $475.00
    Single session videos available (each tape includes 5 guides) .... each $95.00
      Session 1: Lifestyle / Session 2: Eating / Session 3: Exercise / Session 4:
      Stress / Session 5: Relationships / Session 6: Change

  Managing Job Stress Series (6 videos, Leader & Skill Building Guides) $475.00
    Single session videos available (each tape includes 5 guides) .... each $95.00
      Session 1: Handling Workplace Pressure / Session 2: Clarifying Roles
      and Expectations / Session 3: Controlling the Workload / Session 4:
      Managing People Pressures / Session 5: Surviving the Changing
      Workplace / Session 6: Balancing Work and Home

  Manage It! Series (6 videos, Leader & Skill Building Guides) $475.00
    Single session videos available (each tape includes 5 guides) .... each $95.00
      Session 1: Stress Traps / Session 2: Stress Overload / Session 3:
      Interpersonal Conflict / Session 4: Addictive Patterns / Session 5: Job
      Stress / Session 6: Survival Skills

Team Esteem Series (6 videos, Leader & Skill Building Guides) $475.00
Single session videos available (each tape includes 5 guides) .... each $95.00
    Session 1: Overview: The Team Esteem Difference / Session 2: Team
    Talk / Session 3: Team Energy / Session 4: Team Artistry / Session 5:
    Team Mission / Session 6: Putting Team Esteem to Work

Audio Resources
StressTalk $11.95
Stress Breaks
    BreakTime $11.95
    Natural Tranquilizers $11.95
    Stress Escapes $11.95
    Worry Stoppers $11.95
Daydreams
    Daydreams 1: Getaways $11.95
    Daydreams 2: Peaceful Places $11.95
    Daydreams 3: Relaxing Retreats $11.95
Wilderness Daydreams
    Canoe / Rain $11.95
    Island / Spring $11.95
    Campfire / Stream $11.95
    Sailboat / Pond $11.95
Sensational Relaxation
    Countdown to Relaxation $11.95
    Daybreak / Sundown $11.95
    Take a Deep Breath $11.95
    Relax . . . Let Go . . . Relax $11.95
    Stress Release $11.95
    Warm & Heavy $11.95
Mini Meditations
    Healing Visions $11.95
    Refreshing Journeys $11.95
    Healthy Choices $11.95
Guided Meditation
    Inner Healing $11.95
    Personal Empowering $11.95
    Healthy Balancing $11.95
    Spiritual Centering $11.95
    Mantras $11.95
Do-It-Yourself Relaxation
    Yoga $11.95
    Massage $11.95
Do-It-Yourself Wellness
    Eating $11.95
    Body Image $11.95
    Calm Down $11.95
Relaxation / Meditation Music
    Tranquility $11.95
    Harmony $11.95
    Serenity $11.95
    Contemplation (CD) $15.95

Call 1-800-247-6789 to receive a catalog or to place an order.

**Visit our website at http://www.wholeperson.com/~books to view
all our products or to receive further information.**

218-727-0505 (fax)   books@wholeperson.com (e-mail)

ABOUT WHOLE PERSON ASSOCIATES

At Whole Person Associates we're 100% committed to providing stress and wellness materials that involve participants and provide a "whole person" focus—body, mind, spirit, and relationships.

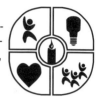

ABOUT THE OWNERS

Whole Person Associates was created by the vision of two people: Donald A. Tubesing, PhD, and Nancy Loving Tubesing, EdD. Don and Nancy have been active in the stress management/wellness promotion movement for over twenty years—consulting, leading seminars, writing, and publishing. Most of our early products were the result of their creativity and expertise. Living proof that you can "stay evergreen," Don and Nancy remain the driving force behind the company and are still very active in developing new products that touch people's lives.

ABOUT THE COMPANY

Whole Person Associates was "born" in Duluth, Minnesota, and we remain committed to our lovely city on the shore of Lake Superior. We put the same high quality into every product we offer, translating the best of current research into practical, accessible, easy-to-use materials. We create the best possible resources to help our customers teach about stress management and wellness promotion. And our friendly and resourceful employees are committed to helping you find the products that fit your needs.

We also strive to treat our customers as we would like to be treated. If we fall short of our goals in any way, please let us know.

ABOUT OUR ASSOCIATES

Who are the "associates" in Whole Person Associates? They're the trainers, authors, musicians, and others who have developed much of the material you see on these pages. We're always on the lookout for high-quality products that reflect our "whole person" philosophy and fill a need for our customers. Our products were developed by experts who are at the top of their fields, and we're very proud to be associated with them.

ABOUT OUR CUSTOMERS

We'd love to hear from you! Let us know what you think of our products—how you use them in your work, what additional products you'd like to see, and what shortcomings you've noted. Write us or call on our toll-free line. We look forward to hearing from you!

**Call 1-800-247-6789 to receive a catalog
or to place an order. Or visit our website at
http://www.wholeperson.com/~books**